TURNING
PAIN
INTO
STRENGTH

BY **MICHELLE EBERWEIN**

Copyright

E-BOOK ISBN: 978-1-7370906-0-1
PAPERBACK ISBN: 978-1-7370906-1-8

Author & Publisher
Michelle Eberwein
TurningPainIntoStrength.com

Co-Author & Editor
Lauren Love BWCopy.com

Logo & Cover Designer
Anatolios Spyrlidis
AnatolioSpyrlidis.com

Appreciation

ROB, MY HUSBAND

Thank you, Rob, my best friend, and soulmate. Without your constant encouragement and support, I would never have had the courage to write this book or finish it. I love you.

KYLE & KANE, MY BOYS

Kyle and Kane, thank you for always being there for me and being the best part of my days! Thank you for letting me be your imperfect mom. I love you both more than words could ever say.
You are my world.

LAUREN, MY CO-AUTHOR

Thank you to my Co-Author and Editor, Lauren, for your ongoing patience. More importantly, for sticking by me while this book took just a tad longer than we expected. Thank you for putting my story into words and for being a special part of my journey.

Contents

Author's Note

'PAIN IS MY DRIVING FORCE'

My life changed forever when I tripped on a step in my basement. It is hard to accept that things will never be the same again.

Relentless chronic pain, a life-threatening addiction to pharmaceutical drugs, surgeries, and surgical disasters have all played a consistent role in my life since the accident happened. This book is about my journey through it all, the inspiring highs, torturous lows, and how I escaped the reigns of medical addiction. It has taken me over a decade to build the knowledge I possess now; knowledge that I feel is invaluable to every human being on this planet, regardless of health. I understand what severe depression and chronic loneliness can do to a person's mind. I experienced, firsthand, the corruption inside our 'healthcare' system.

But no longer do I spend my days feeling like a burden or wishing I were dead. I broke the chains of addiction and graduated as a Certified Medical Assistant, Nutrition and Health Coach. By learning the medical field and the benefits of good nutrition, combined with everything I learned at Rehab concerning self-healing and natural pain management, I have the tools to manage my pain without the need for regular high doses of strong medication.

As a nation, we have become so reliant on a profit-driven medical system to take care of us during our times of need.

- Why are we not taught about the power of good nutrition and self-healing at school?
- Why are free, natural remedies, not promoted as options alongside prescribed medications?

Today, I wake up feeling grateful to be alive. Life can change in the blink of an eye, but it is how you handle the change that matters. Channel your pain to build strength and use that strength to nurture your mind. Isolation, addiction, depression, and helplessness do not have to be a part of your journey. Know that suicide is not an option; I am here for you. The most powerful freedom I have experienced is when I stopped caring about the opinions of others and acted to selfheal through understanding the psychology of self.

Although different, you can still have a life and live it. Living in a permanent state of numbness is not the way out, as we cannot heal if we cannot feel.

Michelle Eberwein

Certified Medical Assistant
Certified Holistic Health & Pain Coach

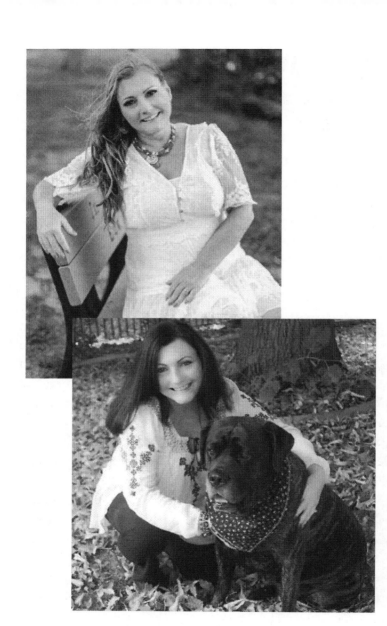

CHAPTER 1

Life Force

As much as we like to believe we control our lives, no one is free from the risk of an accident happening. My life changed forever in 2006. Today, I wake up feeling grateful to be alive.

My name is Michelle Eberwein. I'm from Chicago, Illinois.

I have been happily married to my husband since the age of eighteen. Rob has always been a kind and loving influence in my life, my rock through thick and thin. Together, we have two handsome boys, Kyle (26) and Kane (24). We are a close-knit family and have always encouraged the boys to partake in sporting activities that play a role in their physical and mental development. Every year, we would faithfully support them in their passion for playing hockey. We spent every weekend traveling to games and tournaments out of state and out of the country. We were always on the go, making snacks and renting DVDs for the long car rides, washing jerseys, packing, and loading the car for yet another hockey weekend.

We would spend hours in the stands watching hockey practices, attend dinner parties, and enjoy drinks with the other parents after the games. I loved every minute of our journeys and the chaos that went with them. I guess you could say that my life felt complete; I was appreciative of what I had. We were a solid unit and had everything we needed for a fun, adventurous lifestyle. As the winter hockey season ended, we were enjoying a break before spring hockey began.

It all happened on a warm afternoon; we were at home, the windows were open, and the boys were playing happily in the driveway. I had decided to start spring-cleaning chores and began by storing all the heavy winter clothes away in the basement. Upstairs, I pulled out the storage bins and filled them to the brim, ready to take downstairs. They were heavy, so I had to drag them behind me, but as I reached the third or fourth step from the bottom, I slipped and fell directly onto my butt. The first thing I did was look around to see if anyone had seen me. If they had, I am sure they would have found it hilarious. I stood up, dusted myself off, and continued to place the bins in the storage room. I had no understanding of what had just happened. A big fat bruise was inevitable, but I had just tripped and rolled directly down the rabbit hole.

That night, I started feeling pains in my lower back.

In the knowledge that I had jarred my body earlier that day, I assumed a muscle had strained, and that the pain would pass. Instead, it got worse, and developed into a sharp shooting pain, spreading viciously down my side and through my right leg. Taking advice from my husband, I finally gave in and agreed to seek medical advice. I booked an appointment with our family doctor and informed him about what had happened. He carried out a few tests and reassured me that there was *"absolutely nothing to worry about."* He then prescribed me Vicodin and muscle relaxers to 'help me heal'.

Across the US, prescribed pain relief medication plays a role in many lives. However, it does not provide a solution in most cases. Numbing your pain over long periods can impact negatively on your body's natural processes. How can you heal from the pain if you cannot feel it? By continuing to take pain meds daily, all you are doing is masking the problem instead of fixing it, which can then lead to various other underlying health issues developing, including anxiety, depression, and addiction.

Regardless of the rapidly increasing addiction and mental health issues surrounding pain medications, our healthcare system still fails to provide us with other options and refuses to advise us on free and natural healing methods, which are readily available to all. Of course, pain medication will always seem to be the most appealing option because it guarantees instant relief. Would you decline something that guarantees to numb your pain? None the wiser, I accepted the Vicodin and relaxers and left his office feeling satisfied that there was, 'absolutely nothing to worry about'. Adopting a positive mindset, I ignored my intuition and chose to believe the 'expert' medical opinion I had received.

But as the weeks passed, the pain got even worse.

As the pain became more and more unbearable, the medication became less and less effective. I was beginning to think that something more serious was going on and remember turning to my husband and saying, half-jokingly, *"Rob, my back hurts so bad, I think it is broken."* We instantly agreed it was time to get a second opinion and booked another appointment with our family doctor.

I went to the appointment with my son, Kane, who was aged nine at the time. The doctor ordered an x-ray of my lower spine and escorted us from his office to the Radiology Department, where the x-ray was taken. This time, the result was quite different.   Usually, after an x-ray is taken, the patient is sent home and instructed to wait for the results. In this case, I was still getting dressed when the nurse hurriedly entered the room. She said that the radiologist needed to see me immediately.

Nothing could have prepared me for what came next. As we sat down, an elderly man dressed in a gray radiology coat walked into the room. He was calm and said, *"I am not supposed to give you any results, Michelle, but it is Easter weekend, and you must know, your back is broken."*

Drifting into a dream-like state, I felt the blood drain away from my face & a tingling went through my body. Surely this could not be real. This could not be me. I am thirtyseven years of age and perfectly healthy!

He reached over and handed me the picture of my x-ray, and there, in its white form, was the L4 vertebra with a clearly defined crack through it. He gave me a set of hard copy films and advised me to see an orthopedic surgeon, right away.

"And be careful," he said. *"You don't want to end up paralyzed."*

My husband, Rob, and I

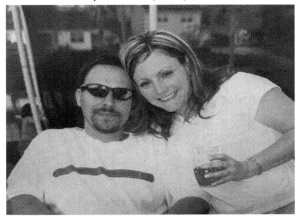

My two boys, Kyle and Kane

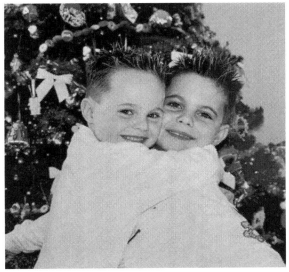

CHAPTER 2

2-Level Disaster

Taking a long, deep breath, I tried everything in my power to hold back the tears. I took my son by the hand and walked out of the doctor's office. Thankfully, he was too young to understand the seriousness of what had just occurred. I was adamant not to cry and put on my best brave act in front of him. However, as we entered the lobby, my self-control escaped me. It was impossible to keep it together as I was petrified about what this meant for our future. As I reached for my cell phone to call Rob, my hands trembled uncontrollably. Repeatedly hitting the wrong numbers, I finally got through. I told him everything!

If there is one thing you should know about my husband, it is that he is the man you need in a crisis, most of the time. Admittedly, he is not particularly useful in 'the dog gets sprayed by a skunk crisis,' but definitely in cases relating to bad health news. He has such a calming effect on me and nearly always knows the right thing to say. As I finished telling him about what had happened, he immediately reassured me that we would get through it together. This left me feeling calm enough to drive home safely with my boy. When I returned, I could not take my eyes off the x-rays. I must have looked at them over a hundred times from every angle and under every light.

It was hard to believe that I was looking at MY spine.

There was me thinking the worst-case scenario would be being bedridden for months while the vertebrae healed, but the truth was far worse than what I had assumed it could be. I had just received the most horrific news, and this was just the beginning. The doctor's last words kept repeating in my head:

>*"And be careful, you don't want to end up paralyzed."*
>*"And be careful, you don't want to end up paralyzed."*
>*"And be careful, you don't want to end up paralyzed."*

The following day was my son's hockey game. His best friend was also on the team, and his dad was an orthopedic surgeon. It was the perfect opportunity for me to get another opinion. I hated to bother him at a hockey rink on his day off, but I felt scared and desperate. When we arrived, I asked him if he would look at my x-rays. He took them to the window of the hockey rink and held them up to the light. I remember how quickly he turned around to confirm if they were *my* x-rays. *"Michelle, you need to be in my office first thing on Monday morning. Your back is fractured. You need to have this taken care of, right away!"* he told me.

I spent the rest of the weekend taking Vicodin and muscle relaxers to try and ease the pain, but nothing was working.

My fear of the unknown was beginning to consume me.

The following Monday morning, I arrived at his office for a meeting with the spine specialist. I walked in with my x-rays in hand and no clue about what to expect. He confirmed what we already knew and ordered an MRI Scan (Magnetic Resonance Imaging) to look at the spinal cord and assess the discs in between the vertebrae. He instructed me to return two weeks later for the MRI results and increased my dosage of Vicodin to further ease the pain.

After two long weeks of hoping and praying, I returned to his office for my results. The MRI report showed that I was already suffering from Degenerative Disc Disease, which meant I had no cushion in between my lumbar vertebrae. When I fell, they cracked against each other, causing one of the discs to rupture.

It was a 2-level disaster.
L3-L4 had broken, and L4-L5 had too.

According to the spine specialist, the only way to fix this injury was to have Spinal Fusion Surgery. A Spinal Fusion is where the surgeon removes what remains of the discs, inserts synthetic bone material as a replacement, and uses screws and rods to stabilize the spine until new bone grows around the vertebrae, to 'fuse' it. It sounds smart and impressive until you visualize the process happening to you. I thought this spine doctor must be a quack or surgery-happy because there was no way I was going to go for it! I had never broken any bones or had surgery before in my life. WHY was this happening to me now?

I could not accept surgery as the only solution. My husband and I continued our research and sought out another spine doctor; there had to be another way to fix this mess. He suggested trying all the conventional methods but stated that, eventually, I would have to have the surgery.

Hockey season was just around the corner, and despite my condition, I carried on as per usual. As a mother, I vowed to always put my children's needs before my own. I decided against the surgery and opted for a course of strong pain medication, antiinflammatories, and muscle relaxers to help me through our journey. I also scheduled my first epidural injection to numb the nerves in my back that were causing me pain. I believed I was doing the right thing for my family and allowing myself more time to learn about all the available options.

This injury has forced me to make decisions I never thought I would have to make in my lifetime. Nobody wants to be a burden on their family and friends. If you had asked me then, I was sure I had made the right decision, replacing surgery with pain medication.

Growing up close to my grandmother taught me about courage. She inspired me to fight the demons obscuring my path through life and always encouraged me to never give up. As a young girl, she too suffered a serious back injury that caused her problems for the rest of her life. In all my memories of her, she never exposed her emotional struggles to anyone. Only now do I realize how much strength she was generating to keep her smile. There was a life lesson to be learned from this phenomenal woman; she became my reason for fighting.

During my monthly meetings with the spine doctor, we tried new treatments, injections, medications, and virtually anything to keep me off that operating room table. I also tried Lidocaine patches, physical therapy, essential oils, heating pads, and ice packs. The pain was soul-destroying, and there is nothing I would not have tried. It was not long before the spine doctor suggested I see a pain management doctor for a stronger and more instant pain relief option.

*"**He will have the good stuff**,"* he said.

I still clutch desperately to my belief that everything happens for a reason and that self-doubt is a journey I do not wish to embark on. Of course, there have been challenging periods where I have allowed this psyche to escape me, but somehow, I always attract it back again. I convinced myself that I was the strong woman I had always been and promised myself never to let my family down. My husband worked so hard to support us, and our boys deserved a strong and active mother to support them. I needed pain relief to make sure I could go on being that mother. I was not going to allow my pain to get in the way of anything.

As always, I attended the games with my family, but it was not the wisest decision I have ever made. Booking myself in for surgery and preventing further deterioration would have been better. My logic or yours; it is all the same language when you are not thinking straight.

Ironically, throughout the games, it was obvious to my husband and sons that I was suffering. I was in so much pain that I no longer even appeared to be the strong and reliable wife and mother I was hoping to achieve. There is an exceptionally fine line between being honest and putting on a façade for the world to see. The people closest to you will most likely know what the right decision is for you. Upon arriving home after the season ended, my family persuaded me to book a date for surgery.

The more I thought about it, the worse I felt. However, I considered myself incredibly lucky to be covered under my husband's health insurance policy. The doctor's appointments, pain medication, therapy, and injections, were getting costly. Without Rob's health insurance, we would never have been able to afford them.

Surgery was scheduled for March 2007.

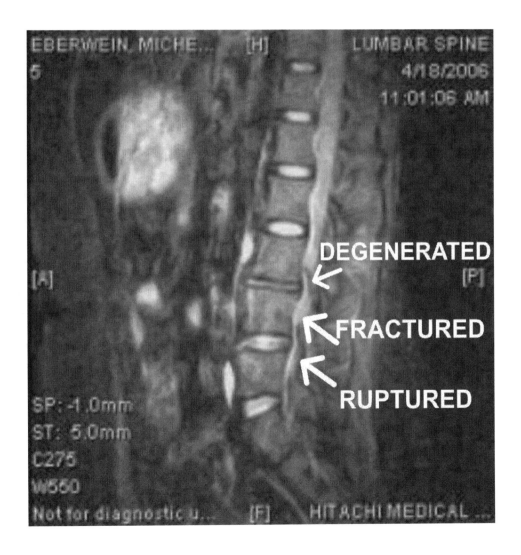

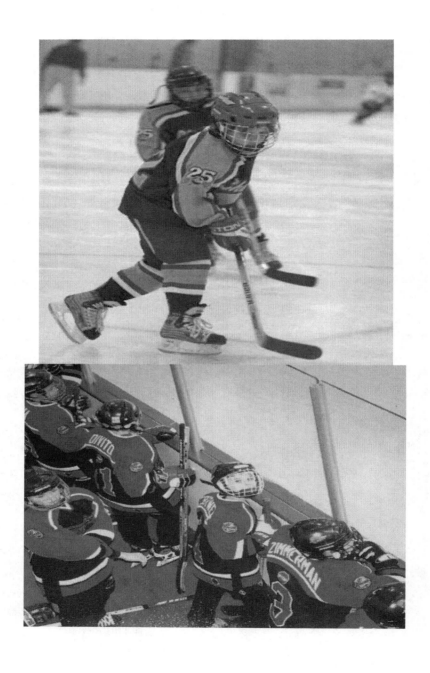

CHAPTER 3

Close Call

The months leading up to my surgery were challenging to say the least! The pain meds were no longer working and basic everyday movements such as getting dressed, walking, and sitting, were becoming impossible for me to do alone. I could barely even carry myself to the bathroom when I needed to. The agony had me constantly wondering whether I would ever walk again, let alone whether I would ever work again. I often thought about how lucky I was to have such a loving family and support circle around me and was always grateful to my husband for his occupation, which guaranteed my medical insurance.

Then, one day, after nineteen consecutive years working for the same company, my husband became unemployed. He arrived at work one morning to find everything closed – shut down. There was no sign of the employers, no communication lines open, and no more Insurance Plan covering me. The company had gone bust, and a hefty one-hundred-and-thirty-thousand-dollar medical bill (which was about to rise significantly a few weeks later) became our responsibility.

Powerlessness and guilt are two of the best words I can use to describhow I felt. There was nothing I could do to help the situation, and watching my husband be so worried about how to support us was difficult for me. The more I thought about the future, the more I realized the long-term effects my injury could have on all of us.

Becoming a slave to the system that rules you is a nightmare that peoplincreasingly face, and the outcome is rarely positive. Surgery was getting closer, the pain was intensifying, and it was time my husband and I joined forces to combat these issues together. We vowed to keep matters of financial stress away from the boys and made a joint decision to file for bankruptcy.

Mentally, I was all over the place. I was worried about the surgery going wrong but also felt excited at the thought of returning to a life without pain. Part of my mind was completely numb from the side effects of the medication, while another part was frantically digging for strength to help me prepare for the big day. Keeping myself calm and level-headed was a huge challenge that I was struggling to beat. I would constantly tell myself that I was strong and that everything was going to run smoothly, but the Sword of Damocles was hanging over me. I was secretly terrified. I applied for state-funded health insurance, and, thankfully, it was approved one week before the date of surgery.

When the day finally arrived, I felt hopeful that it would bring an end to all my pain. The medical staff were extremely friendly and came across as professionals you could rely on for honest medical guidance. I asked them how long the surgery was expected to last and received a confident response from one of the nurses, who said, *"4-6 hours from start to finish."* I decided this was good news and convinced myself that it could have been a lot worse. I tried not to think about the one-year recovery period that was to follow. It was time to embrace my surroundings, hand myself over to the 'medical experts', and hope for the best.

The nurse handed me a hospital gown, and everyone left the room while I changed. As I slowly undressed, I felt my mindset slipping into a much darker place. I pictured my little boy's faces when I left the house that morning; they had tears running down their cheeks. I could not help but think about what would happen to them if the surgery went wrong. What would happen if they were left with no mother to take care of them? How could I leave my husband to raise them alone? Then, I started thinking gruesome thoughts about the surgical process and how I was about to have my stomach cut wide open and organs removed. How was I supposed to know if I was making the right decision? I put on the gown, and we continued.   It was, by no means, a smooth start. After twelve failed attempts by the nurses to put a needle in my arm for IV treatment, the anesthesiologist was called in. They finally managed to reach a vein, but the pain was intolerable by that point. The surgery had not even started, and I had tears pouring down my face. They supplied me with a concoction of what they called *'calming meds'* and prompted me to say *'goodbye'* to my husband, mom, and sister. What the hell was I supposed to be thinking by this point? I tried hard to control my nerves and was wheeled routinely into the operating room. I remember the temperature drop to ice-cold, the shiny steel tools positioned militarily across the surfaces, and the bright white floodlights suspended directly above the bed. I felt my chest tightening up.

Then, I drifted.

It sounds so cliché, but I have vivid memories of floating down a tunnel of brilliant white light. No fear, no pain; it was just how some movies depict death, and it felt like a peaceful place to be. I felt warm, safe, and free. I have no idea how long those feelings lasted but I do remember waking up. As I regained consciousness, the surge of pain that followed was indescribable. I screamed out loud. I could see the nurses walking around, talking to each other, and laughing, but no one heard me. I screamed again as the pain just about ripped me in half, and the nurses came running. I remember the shock on their faces as they approached my bed.

"What's the matter?" they asked.

"I think I'm dying. My heart is beating so hard in my chest! Am I OK?" I responded frantically.

Suddenly, I was surrounded by medical staff and, then came the syringe. I drifted once more. Everything slowed down after that, and my next memory is being wheeled down the hallway on my bed. I remember seeing my husband's face and feeling safe knowing that he was there with me, but the questions in my mind were racing. What happened during my surgery? Why is my mom crying like that? Where is my sister, and why is she not

23

yelling at her to stop? Why is my heart beating so fast? How are my children? Where are they taking me? Am I dying?

It turns out that the surgery did not last for four or six hours. Instead, it had taken thirteen hours to complete! My husband told me that I needed a blood transfusion. I also found out that after a cut iliac artery and a fifteen-inch abdominal incision, I had just survived a *"very close call".* The blood transfusion was required to stop me from dying soon after the surgery.

They informed me that it would only be several days before I could return home. A part of me was too weak to care about anything, but the good news of returning home gave me the boost I needed to keep going. My mom, sister, and my beloved husband stayed by my side and were able to make the medical decisions I could not. I remember watching the blood empty from the bag, flow down the tube, and into my arm. Getting someone else's blood put into your body is a very strange feeling; a feeling that I did not know I would experience again, later in life. The days following the blood transfusion had me focused on building up energy, and mentally preparing for the recovery period ahead. Every day, my medical team got me out of bed, walked me with my walker, and sat me up in a chair, but something did not feel right. I was still so weak, and my heart was beating at such a rapid pace.

Was I experiencing the usual side effects of post major surgery?

After a long week in the hospital, the nurses sent me home in a thick hard plastic cast, fixed from just under my breasts, down to my hips. I also had a walker, but I barely had the strength to use it alone. The pain was intense, but the excitement to get home and see my boys was much stronger.

The day I returned to my comfort zone was the day I felt grateful for everything I had. I refused to let the pain get me down and felt safe, in the knowledge that a Home Health Nurse was appointed to visit me daily. The purpose of her visit was to ensure my recovery was progressing smoothly and that I was not being severely affected by any abnormal side effects. During the visits, I was urged to discuss any queries I had, and to request professional help in areas where I was unable to function without assistance. Everything was beginning to look rosy for the first time in a while. Surgery was over, and I believed this was a sign of good things to come. I told myself that once the recovery period was also over, my life would go back to normal. I had to control my emotions if I wanted to walk again.

It felt good to have such a supportive family, and I was thankful to my mom, who had left my dad and her dog in Florida, to move in with us. She stayed for four months during my recovery and helped readjust my home so that everything was positioned at waist height. This was because I was unable to bend, lift, or twist. She washed me, dressed me, and carried out household chores that I was unable to do. If I dropped something on the floor, someone nearby would have to pick it up for me. I could not even hug my children without pain interfering.

It was not long before I started to feel like a burden on all of themMentally, this presented a dangerous crossing-point because although I believed that my family would be better off without me, the reality was quite different. Feeling like a burden led me into a dark and lonely headspace, where self-value was non-existent. It was not until years later that I realized I was never a burden at all. It was my perception that was warped, and my mindset was just a reflection of that.

After a week of being back at home, I noticed a strange lump appear in my arm, in the same place where the IV line had been connected. I mentioned it to my home nurse when she arrived later that afternoon. She sent me to the ER for a series of tests to be carried out, and the results showed a blood clot in my arm where the lump was visible. I was informed that an overnight stay was required in the hospital to monitor the blood clot and reduce the risk of infection. That is the last thing I wanted to hear, but I convinced myself that one more night was doable. I accepted the doctor's instruction and was directed to my room. Deep down, I was devastated to be back in hospital again. I focused my energy on getting through the night without crumbling.

I had finally gotten comfortable when my evening took a lethal turn. Before nightfall, on the same day, I was further diagnosed with pneumonia. Having a weakened immune system was starting to trigger infections in my body, and my recovery seemed to be moving further and further away. Determined not to let it get the better of me, I refused to give in to self-pity and fear.

I took a pain pill and drifted back to my familiar state of numbness.

CHAPTER 4

Unsolicited Shutdown

Returning home to my family was everything to me, and I was so pleased to be out of that clinical environment. Although difficult, I had no choice but to focus my mind and prepare for the recovery period once more. Following the surgery, I was prescribed Morphine, to ease the pain while my body healed. It was not an easy way to live, but how could I go on feeling sorry for myself when I had such an amazing family? How could I not be grateful for the loving energies helping me every day? Where would I be right now without them?   All was going well until five days later when my body started rejecting all food and liquid. The pain increased ferociously. I had no understanding of what was happening to me and remember being frightened for my life. Why could I not hold anything down? Why was the pain getting worse this time? Hesitantly, I made another call to our family doctor and arranged yet another appointment at his earliest convenience. He advised that the rejection of food was a direct result of the high levels of pain I was suffering, and prescribed Fentanyl patches on top of the Morphine I had already received, postoperatively, from the neurosurgeon.

"This should help relieve your pain," he said.

Financial gain for the pharmaceutical industry should never be the driving force in any medical strategy. Have you ever wondered why doctors do <u>not</u> inform us about free and natural healing methods?   None the wiser, I trusted his professional opinion and hoped that soon, his guidance would save me from this ongoing nightmare.

I was beginning to feel defeated and was struggling to keep a positive mindset. The moment you allow your mind to slip into a negative downhill spiral, you will learn that getting it back can be tough. The struggle was real, every single day, and the pain was becoming a prominent part of my life. I knew I was becoming addicted to pharmaceutical drugs because I was willing to try anything if it meant numbing the pain, as well as my brain.

When I got home, I applied the newly prescribed Fentanyl patches to help manage the severe agony I was experiencing. To begin with, I felt drowsy, and within the hour, I was practically asleep; I could not stay awake. Being asleep meant that I could not feel pain, and that was what I wanted. Being awake was exhausting! Moving, speaking, and even the act of breathing had become painful.

A whole day had passed before I finally woke up again. My mom was next to me, trying to feed me soup, but I could not even keep that down. As soon as anything hit my stomach, my body was triggered to vomit. She insisted on calling the doctor who prescribed a further course of anti-nausea pills, but nothing helped. The vomiting was constant, and dehydration was becoming yet another issue I had to deal with. Two days later, I still had not eaten. I got out of bed to go to the bathroom; the entire room started to spin.

I fainted.

When I finally regained consciousness, I could not breathe. My heart was pounding so violently in my chest that I could hear it echoing in my ears. I was crying but there were no tears. Severe dehydration was beginning to affect my body, and I was in a state of utter confusion. How long was I gone for? Why can I not move my legs? What is happening? Do I need to go back to the hospital? Please, no! Why? Am I dying?

My mom was still there, by my side, and gave me an ultimatum. *"You either get in the car, or I am calling an ambulance. You are going to the hospital, Michelle!"* she said firmly. She was concerned about me and adamant that I went for help. I have little memory of getting in the car and being driven there. Everything was blurry, and I could barely speak. All I wanted to do was sleep. My energy had evaporated. I had no fight left in me. My mom did most of the talking when we arrived, and the doctor ordered tests to find out what was going on.

Then, I drifted.

Waking up in the hospital was nothing new by this point. The doctors informed me that I had suffered respiratory distress and that my digestive system had shut down. The cause was the Fentanyl patches I had been prescribed to take with the Morphine and Oxycodone that I was already taking! Putting it simply, my doctor had led me to overdose on pharmaceutical drugs, which resulted in an unsolicited shutdown of my entire mind and body. I was officially guided over the edge - by a medical professional. I was lucky to be alive.

It was not the first time I had survived a close call. A further four days of recovering in the hospital was not going to bring me down. It gave me time to think about what had happened.

How should I have felt? Furious at the doctor for leading me to overdose and nearly ending my life? Happy about the fact I was still alive? In all honesty, I was livid but had to dig deep if I wanted to recover. The doctor said the patches must have been defective and possibly dispensing more Fentanyl than designed too. I will never know. I wanted to channel my focus onto brighter things, and within a few days, I was beginning to feel better. My confidence levels rose as I thought more and more about the future. Surely nothing else could go wrong after what I had been through. I could not allow anger to get in the way of my healing.

Was I on the road to recovery this time? Could I finally heal and move forward in life? I could barely walk, but I could see a subtle hint of hope lurking in my peripheral vision. I used that hope to guide me through the following months after the overdose, but it did not last for as long as I had hoped it would.

My addiction to pain meds was becoming a problem that I could no longer ignore. I was fully aware of the side effects taking place and lived in an altered state of consciousness – all the time. It was a warm and fuzzy feeling with much less pain! I had lost interest in pretty much everything and had developed a switch to control my headspace. Around my family, it was ON, and the rest of the time, it was OFF, which proved to be a very lonely and profound place to be. As the months passed, I was slowly switching OFF around my family too.

My life seemed to mirror that of my grandmother' more and more. The only difference is that I gradually became wholly detached. The control I had over my emotional switch was lost, and I was encroaching into a zone of ultimate depression. Being unable to move freely around your home and carry out the most basic of household chores becomes very frustrating. They had removed the Fentanyl from my prescription, but I was still taking Morphine and Oxycodone to help manage the post-surgical pain. They were keeping me up all night and into the early hours of the morning. I could not sleep. I would sit on the couch after everyone had gone to bed and feel an imaginary but warm presence, like a blanket, wrap itself around me as the pain medication traveled through my body. The darkness and silence of the room permitted me to feel comfortably numb, without the need to feel guilty or act bravely around anyone. I was wide awake. I wanted to give up. I did not have the strength to fight anymore. The pain was exhausting. My kids were always *"worried about mommy,"* and my husband was under a lot of stress. Nobody should have to endure so much pain in such a short period. I was done!

Fiddling with the bottle of pain medications, night after night, thinking about how many it would take to put me to sleep forever. If I were to put an end to my life, what impact would it have on my family? Rob would need to take the boys shopping to buy suits for the funeral, while he would probably wear his brown suit. I researched the price of caskets and considered my funeral costs. The last thing I wanted to do was leave them with more financial burdens and unnecessary debt. A vivid mental image of myself, lying peacefully in a casket, in no pain, remains with me today. That is all I wanted; to be free of pain.

It was not the first time I had visualized myself lying in a casket. When I was sixteen, I endured a long period of emotional and psychological struggle. It was different from the physical pain I later faced. I remember removing the lid from a bottle of sleeping pills and washing every single one of them down with red wine. I was so young and desperate to put an end to the torture. Fortunately, it was not my time to leave. I woke up in the Intensive Care Unit having my stomach pumped. They then sent me to a Treatment Center where they supervised me daily for three months. Looking back, it was a good time for contemplation, and I learned a lot about myself from that experience.   But this time was different. I could feel myself losing control of my thoughts until suddenly, I began thinking about my grandmother. How did she uphold her courage for so many years? How did she control the pain and still lead a normal life? I followed my intuition and took these questions as a sign to call her. When she answered, the sound of her voice instantly calmed me. I explained how pain and fear were ruling my life, and how suicidal thoughts were slowly taking over. I should have known what response I would get, but I needed to hear it from her.

"To even consider leaving your children and husband is wrong, no matter how you feel, Michelle. Knock it off!" she responded abruptly.

Just by reaching out to her and making that call, I released myself from the dark pit I was festering in. Her words have stuck with me since that day and inspired me in the most challenging of circumstances. I decided I wanted to achieve the same for my boys that my grandmother did around me as a child. She became my driving force, and I started believing that if grandma could do it smiling, so could I.

By the summer of 2007, glimpses of hope for a healthy future were making appearances. Medication was still a part of my life, but I felt hopeful that this would change. Physically, I was getting stronger, so my surgeon appointed a physical therapist to guide me in strengthbuilding.

It was the beginning of a new chapter for me – a fresh challenge that required me to step out of my comfort zone and switch ON again. My husband was happy to be back in employment, my boys were content, and I was ready to embrace whatever I had to do to get better.

According to the surgeon, it was time to build physical strength.

CHAPTER 5

Wealth for Health

My lifestyle was improving, and I appreciated every move I was able to make. Albeit slow, excellent progress was being made. It felt so good to be moving again and I was proud of myself for what I had achieved. Was I finally moving out of the dark and into the light? I often think about how I took my limbs for granted before I lost use of them. It is hard to describe the feeling of living in a state where your mind is functioning, but your body is not.

My newly appointed physical therapist created a fitness program tailored to my medical history and strength levels. Of course, I doubted any so-called expert advice that came my way. I was cynical but decided to trust her professional guidance. In hindsight, I should have gone with my gut!

She became a motivational factor in my supportive circle and focused the fitness plan on strengthening my stomach muscles, which had been cut open by the surgeon to access my spinal cord. Overwhelming feelings of confidence and self-esteem were creeping back into my existence, and the more I was able to move, the happier I became. The effects of physical training on your mental balance are unbeatable. I felt physically and mentally stronger!

One afternoon, however, I arrived for my PT session, and things did not go to plan. I started by going through the motions according to the program. My therapist praised me for making good progress and instructed me to begin small sit-ups. I felt immediately apprehensive because I believed it was still too soon after the operation to be doing sit-ups. I raised the concern with her, but she persuaded me that I was ready and that everything was going to be fine.

I ignored my intuition, again, and trusted her specialist guidance like a true optimist.

Halfway through the sit-ups, I stopped suddenly as a sharp pulling sensation took over. Fear rushed through my entire body like a needle in my heart. I informed her that something was not right, gathered my things, and headed home. As I walked hastily out of the rehabilitation center, I could not stop thinking about the worst. I knew I should not have done those 'small' sit-ups. What was I thinking? Had I lost control of my mind? Was I that crazy to consciously ignore my gut instinct and do something I did not feel comfortable doing? It turns out, I was. The worst was far worse than what I had anticipated the worst could be.

I returned home and got undressed to take a shower. As I looked down, a large bulge was sticking out from my incision; it was the size of an orange! I became paralyzed with fear. My mind was racing, and my heart felt as if it was going to bounce out of my chest. I immediately called my mother, petrified for my life. *"What the living hell can this be?"* I asked frantically after explaining what had happened. She told me it sounded like an incisional hernia, in which case, I needed to go to the ER as soon as possible. I felt queasy, scared, and helpless as I contemplated my next move. I called my sister to watch my boys and waited impatiently for my husband to get home from work. I could not help but feel guilty; I dreaded him walking through the door expecting a nice quiet evening after a hard day's work, only to be told I needed to go to the ER, again.

As he arrived home, off we went. I received immediate medical attention and was sent for a CT scan almost instantly. It was an incisional hernia; my mom was right. The movement of sit-ups had caused the incision to tear open on the inside of my stomach, causing my intestines to push out against my skin. I had no words, but I knew this meant one sure thing - more surgery. There I was, back in the deepest of troughs, with the universe closing in on me again. I could not face another surgery, but I had no choice. The only way to get through it was to embrace it. I gave myself 'preparation time' beforehand, which helped me a lot, and gave me more confidence.

My idea of 'preparation time' involves thinking hard about my state of awareness, guiding it to be strong, and having regular pep talks with myself to 'just do it.' Do not focus on how weak you feel, but instead think about how strong you want to be. Focus on the goal instead of the process. Make a conscious deal with yourself to keep a good spirit. When panic sets in, you have got to keep your part of the deal. It is just as important to feel mentally ready, as it is to feel physically ready.

I put off the surgery for a few days while I composed myself. I had to convince myself that I could go through with it, and said, repeatedly, *"It's just one more thing. One more surgery. You can do this!"* My mom agreed to move back into our home once more to look after the boys during my upcoming recovery period. I have no idea how I would have managed without my mom. She enabled my boys to still live a fairly normal life where they were able to continue eating homemade meals, playing hockey, and going to school. This brought me a sense of security and helped me feel calm amidst the chaos.

Surgery day arrived.

All I wanted to do was run away, but deep down, I knew there was no turning back. I was terrified of the unknown and more unpredictable complications occurring. I was informed that the process involved placing a patch over a hole in my abdominal muscles, little incisions, and, yes, more pain. I was taken to a presurgical room and handed a gown.

Taking off my clothes and putting on a surgical gown makes me feel vulnerable, and that is when fear takes over. Reality kicks in as I hand over my fate to the medical 'experts.' The nurse was there with the IV and a sedative to calm my uncontrollable shaking. I was then seated in a wheelchair, wheeled down the hall, and into the operating room. The big and very bright white light was positioned over the bed, and the shiny steel tools were neatly arranged on the table, waiting to be used on me.

Then, I drifted.

I remember waking up in the recovery room and being told that *"everything went well."* According to the surgeon, the reason for the tear was due to *"too much strain on the stomach muscles."* He refused to acknowledge that the damage was caused by the physical therapy guidance I had been receiving and insisted that the muscles were simply *"too weak"* and *"just tore"* because of *"too much strain."*

I soon learned that everyone in the medical profession protects each other. I knew the truth but had no way of proving it. I felt completely deflated, bewildered, and part of me was angry at my physical therapist for encouraging me to do sit-ups at such an early stage in the program. My surgeon's words hit a nerve, and a small but powerful spirit perked up from within me. It was time to fight for my right to receive honest medical guidance. I began investigating and made complaints to the relevant bodies regarding what had happened. I received advice from reliable legal sources, and the general answer went something like, *"you have a strong case here Mrs. Eberwein, but it will be a very costly and drawn-out process."*

Another dead end.

I was left weak and disabled, with a strong case, swimming in debt, and with no affordable support system accessible for me to exercise my right to justice. Eventually, forced to surrender due to lack of funds, I struggled to grasp the idea that you need financial wealth to pay for your health. I no longer had faith in humanity, the legal system, medical experts, or the rest of them; I had no idea where to turn to. I was being swallowed up by the system, and there was no escape.

I was happy when spending time with my family, but the rest of my life was forming a severe state of glumness controlled by my endless supply of loyal pain meds - keeping me balanced nicely on the edge. Despite my attempts to avoid feeling like a burden, it was becoming impossible in my mind to feel any other way. My boys were always taking care of me with ice packs and heating pads. Rob was always stressed because of the pressure it was putting on the family and our relationship. He spent so much of his time wondering when the next complication would arise or when the next ER visit would crop up, and at the same time, he was left with the responsibility of supporting us financially. My mother was taking a lot of time out of her own life to help me with the boys and around the house. It was exhausting for all of us! How could anyone in my shoes **not** feel like a burden?

Complexity, in our minds, is often created by a lack of effective communication, and a sheer lack of knowledge about how our psyche works things out. You can rest assured that the build-up of non-communicated emotions will lead to the birth of a monster.

I chose to hide my feelings and frustrations because I knew that my family was unaware of what I was really going through. I did not want sympathy or help; I just wanted to feel normal again; I wanted to feel alive again; I wanted to be useful again.

I wanted to be ME, again.

My scars form the roadmap of my life. They do not remind me of the pain I once felt, but of how strong I am, never to have given up.

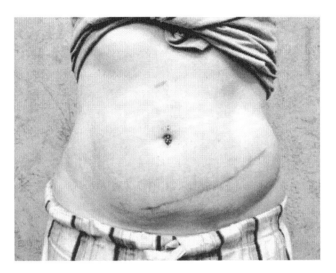

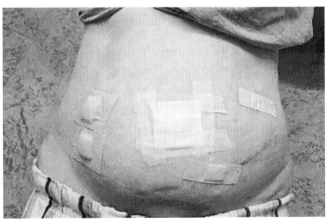

CHAPTER 6
Groundhog Day

By 2008, I no longer felt so alone and had found ways to communicate better with my family and friends. It had finally become clear that no one could read my mind and that I needed to speak up more to help them to understand me. I also had to stop assuming I knew what they were thinking; imagining scenarios based on how I thought they felt about me is one of the very things that led me to feel like a burden. I later learned that my family did not view me as useless or weak, as I did myself, but wanted the best for me. I learned how to explain myself better when I was hurting or when I suddenly needed to lie down. I learned to listen to them without passing judgment or taking offense. By making a conscious effort to connect with them, things gradually started to get easier, and I no longer felt so isolated.

Pent-up emotions can lead to frustration and uncertainty for everyone around you. Frustration then leads to misunderstanding, which can result in self-doubt, anger, and isolation. Feeling isolated can become very lonely and make you incredibly weak. It is a vicious cycle that only you can control.

Find a way to communicate with your loved ones, and if that is not an option for you, remember that I am here. I want to talk to you. From experience, I know exactly how you feel and want to help you. I was still using pain medication, but it was nowhere near as bad as before. A new physical therapist got appointed for me, and as you can imagine, I doubted absolutely everything she advised me to do.

I researched her 'professional' guidance and was extremely careful not to overdo my movements.

One afternoon, during a weekend hockey tournament, we had some time to spare in between games. We started walking and came across a pet store that had my favorite Teacup Yorkie Puppies inside. I wanted one but Rob was not keen on the idea. He agreed to come in and see them with me but insisted that *"the only dog you will walk out of here with is a brindle English Mastiff."* Knowing how rare the English Mastiffs are, we did not expect the pet store to have any, but as we walked in, there she was, a beautiful and lanky awkward-looking Bambi pup, a four-month-old brindle English Mastiff! I took one look at her, and it was love at first sight. I think Rob also went through a series of emotions in a span of a few seconds: shock, disbelief, excitement, and nervousness. Rob knew I was going to want her, but he did not want another dog. We had a black Labrador at home and a cat. My state of health and physical ability restricted the role I could play in her life. This dog was no Teacup Yorkie; this was a big pup!

We were in no position to purchase her right there and then because we had the next hockey game to attend, and, also, Rob did not take it as a sign from above that she was meant to be with us. I had to work on him a little bit. I will never admit that I **may** have called the pet store from the hockey rink bathroom and put a deposit on her with a credit card so that no one could buy her. We picked her up the next day! The staff informed us that we had saved her life, as if we had not taken her, she would have been sent to a shelter the following day. I believe we saved each other.

We were an active hockey family, so we named her Bauer after a popular hockey brand. Over time, I got into the habit of calling her Little Boo, but she was far from little. Eventually, we all called her Boo and only yelled 'BAUER!' when she was caught being mischievous. I will never forget the night we gated her into our hallway and went to bed without realizing that the boys had sneaked her a feather pillow and a blanket for comfort. I woke up to find feathers and fabric everywhere! That was most definitely a 'BAUER!' moment, especially as the pillows had been handed down to me by my grandmother.

On a separate occasion, we had all gone to my grandmother's house for Easter and arrived home to find Boo had escaped her crate. It looked as though a burglary had taken place with thirty pounds of dog food ripped open, half of it eaten, dog food scattered throughout the house, couch pillows torn, the Easter candy, gone, shoes had been chewed to shreds, trophies, hockey pucks, I could go on. She must have gone bananas for six whole hours! My husband walked in through the door behind me, took one look, turned around, walked back out, got into our car, and drove away. That is how destructive my sweet Little Boo was!

We laugh so much about it now, but not on that day.

Boo came with so many trust issues and misbehaved as a result. Trainers would yell at us to *"put her down"* because of a supposed *"mean streak"* she had, but I was not convinced. Deep down, I knew her naughtiness was down to her experience living under a not-so-loving bunch of humans before she came to us. I knew she was not mean; all I could see was an innocent pup that needed love, patience, and time invested in her. I had the time and a lot of love to give.

Giving up was not an option for me. I devoted myself and made it my mission to get her to trust me. I believed that if I could eventually gain her trust, she would feel safe and behave better. It was not long before she settled in and became a solid part of our family unit. Her behavior improved as she adapted to our lifestyle, and, slowly but surely, Boo became the perfect friend. She was always with me and provided me with companionship during my best and darkest moments. I could rely on her to be there when everyone else was busy working or living a normal life. She kept me as active as I could be and provided comforting snuggles whenever I needed them. She became just another reason to smile every day! Looking after Boo and watching her transform into a dutiful and happy house pet was like a dream come true for me. She gave me a sense of achievement and self-worth.

Having a pet can make a significant difference to your well-being and happiness. Unconditional love, regular affection, and constant companionship all come as part and parcel of having a loving pet. Pets do not judge the way you look on those rough days and will loyally stay by your side, no matter what. Cats and dogs are commonly used all over the world as therapy animals. They are used to alleviate stress, anxiety, depression, and feelings of social isolation. Cats are also widely used in prisons to bring comfort to prisoners.

As my health improved, I started attending a new physical therapy center and dedicated myself to a journey of strength-building. Every single day, I fought to keep motivated! My life was getting easier, especially with Boo as my devoted sidekick.

But the unexpected happened again.

After the last surgery, I was told that I could exercise without the risk of another injury happening. Sadly, under the instruction of a different physical therapist, my incisional hernia tore again. It was much worse than the first time and was not supposed to happen in the hands of medical experts. I cannot describe to you how upset I felt. A short glimpse into a happy and healthy life had been shattered, again, and I soon found myself back in the hospital; more surgery was required.

All I could think about was why. Why me, again? I booked an appointment with a different surgeon in a different hospital to find out what was going on. He reckoned that the first hernia patch was not long enough and said the muscles had torn past the patch, causing my intestines to find a way through into the hole, where they became stuck. This was more than just a bad repair job; the previous surgeon had made a terrible mistake in miscalculating the length of the patch.

It was the second surgery for the same injury, but this time it was different. The surgeon had to hand-sew each muscle layer, super tight, to ensure it could never rip again. I gathered up enough energy and courage to ask how long the recovery period would last, and he confirmed, *"four to six weeks."*

Was I supposed to believe him and have faith in what he told me?

I took control of the situation and began preparing for surgery. As usual, I had regular pep talks with myself about staying focused on the goal, not the process. Arrangements were being made for my mom to leave Florida again and move in with us. I had to prepare my kids, my home, and myself. I had to convince myself that I could go through with it and that it would be my last, ever surgery. *"It's just one more thing, one more surgery, Michelle. You can do this!"* I told myself.

When surgery day finally arrived, there was no turning back. I arrived at my appointment feeling hopeful yet angry. I was asked to change into a gown and take a seat in a wheelchair - Groundhog Day. They wheeled me directly to the surgical room. The process and emotions felt all too familiar; I hated it. I was tired of people telling me to *"stay strong,"* and I was no longer keen on *"staying positive"* either. What was the point when bad things kept happening? I was tired of this routine. It was so hard to stay confident when I felt so weak and helpless.

Then, I drifted.

As I regained consciousness, I remember feeling furious. I could not understand why these experts were not being held responsible for my condition. The surgeon was there and told me, *"Everything went well, Michelle, but I had to place a surgical drain into your incision."* Surgical drains are used after some surgeries to ensure blood and fluid do not accumulate under the incision. It was my job to empty the drain as and when it became full. Just the thought of having a tube stuck in my body made me feel nauseous, let alone having to empty it myself! But I had no other choice. It was just another step on a long list of steps that I was being forced to do. I had to empty it approximately five times a day until my body healed. Having to empty a drain full of your own blood, and other bodily fluids is not a task for the faint-hearted! I was too numb with anger and disbelief to care about anything anymore. Another surgery was over, and I was trying my hardest to recover. All of this was due to the previous surgeon miscalculating the length of the patch – I was being made to pay the price.

Four weeks later, I was still struggling with healing. It was the third abdominal surgery I had received in under eighteen months, and my muscles were taking longer and longer to heal. With every surgery, scar tissue grew, and according to the surgeon, it was seriously affecting the healing process. He had cleaned out a lot of the scar tissue from inside my abdomen, but a lot of it had attached to my organs, so he could not remove all of it. He said that it may grow back twice as thick, and he did not want to risk it.

I could feel the negativity taking over fast. Surely, I had some rights in this complicated mess? How could I be repeatedly treated like this by so-called professionals and experts and be expected to be OK with it? I did not know what to do; I just knew that something was wrong, and that justice was not being served. I felt vindicated for having this happen to me again, but instead of allowing myself to fall victim and suffer, I decided to pursue legal action.

My sweet baby Boo!

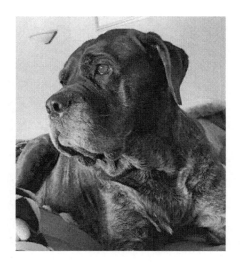

My Boys

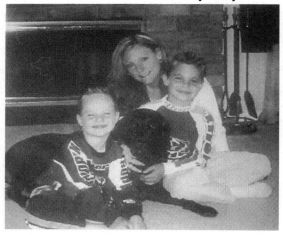

CHAPTER 7

Back to Work

On pain meds, I was living in an altered state of consciousness most of the time. The medication I was taking was so strong that I could barely think straight, let alone find a suitable lawyer. Rob and I carried out internet research, made calls, and sent emails, but not one single lawyer showed interest in my case. Despite our best efforts, we were left powerless and helpless. We found out the hard way just how cruel and deceitful our medical system can be.   It became apparent that doctors act to protect each other and will not disclose evidence if it means harming the reputation or career of another medical professional. Consequently, lawyers in the US prefer not to accept small medical cases like mine, unless it is an open-and-shut case. There were no other options available for me to get justice. I had a hard time accepting that our medical system was so corrupt and profit-driven.

My predicted four-to-six-week recovery turned into ten long weeks. Most of my time was spent in a clouded daze, in bed, with Boo by my side. The days seemed long, the nights, longer, and happiness was a million miles away. Floating in and out of consciousness, I do not know how I would have managed without pain medication. Mentally and physically, I was a mess. It felt like a whole year had passed by the end of the tenth week. My limbs had slowly started to loosen up and moving around was getting easier. It felt so good to be able to move again, but my mind was absent, numb, nobody home.

I was aware that my body was improving, but it was like I had entered some form of mental paralysis. I had given up and there was no more courage left in me to fight and be positive. I could not even find the energy to show affection and love to my family. Everything seemed impossible. All I wanted to do was stay in bed, all day, every day.   I often think about how difficult this was for my husband, mom, and children. Rob, as always, could not do enough to support me. He would come home after a long day's work and sit by my side, to just be with me. I was not a fun person to be around, not active, joyous, and certainly not reliable. I was a zombie.

My family tried to support me by speaking to me and encouraging me to pull through. After a lot of patience and perseverance on their behalf, I eventually began to open up and listen to their words. Rob managed to persuade me that giving up was not an option. His regular reminders to dig deep, find strength, and be confident about my future, started to sink in. Over time, I began to feel again. Rob has always been there when I come out the other side.

"This is your chance to recover fully, Michelle, without any more accidents," he said passionately.

He was right. I had to find a new focus outside of my comfort zone. I battled with my thoughts for quite some time before finally believing in myself again. Having a strong support circle, whether it be two or ten people, is so powerful during times of pain and healing. My mom, husband, sister, and children all played a role in my mental health development and everyday care. I knew I was lucky to have them but also saddened by the thought of others who may not have the same support. I convinced myself that nothing else could go wrong and to trust in my ability to heal.

Towards the end of 2008, I developed strong feelings of gratefulness for what I had in my life. I successfully weaned myself off all prescription pain medications, and my view of the world became clear again.

Do not forget to praise yourself when you deserve it! We are so quick to acknowledge and dwell on our failures that we forget to pat ourselves on the back for all the small steps we take. I was proud of myself for putting a stop to the medication and, by praising myself, contributed to the growth of my self-worth. Why not? It felt good knowing that I had got through it all successfully. My brain was finally given a chance to reset and reformulate before entering back into reality. I knew that I had to stay focused if I was going to get back to normal life. I still had a future to live. I needed a new focus, something to look forward to.

I decided to restart my career as a Certified Nursing Assistant.

Remembering the day that I informed my family I was ready to return to work; they were all so shocked that it made me laugh. My heart has always been set on helping others, and I was so desperate to be useful again. It was not easy, and I did question myself, all the time, about my ability to do it successfully. Doubts regarding my physical ability were always niggling away at me, but once I decided to go for it, there was no turning back.

The job search commenced, and in just a matter of weeks, a job opening popped up with one of the largest medical groups in Illinois. The advert called for a local Home Health Care Nursing Assistant. I could not have wished for a more suitable opportunity, however, there were still questions lingering in the back of my mind. Who would trust an employee with titanium rods and screws in her back? Why would they hire me over and above other, healthier applicants? Would I be able to cope with the workload? What if I was not strong enough? … I took a moment to contemplate my decision, pushed fear aside, and applied for the position. I was invited for an interview just a few days later.

After much consideration, I had decided to omit information relating to past health issues because I knew that it would negatively impact the result of the interview. I was sure that they would not interfere with the job description and felt so good after getting off the meds! If I wanted to get fit again, I had to start feeling it.

I got the job.

By March of 2009, I was busy working as a Home Health Care Nursing Assistant for elderly and disabled patients in my local area. It felt so rewarding to be needed and able to play an active role in the lives of my children, family, and patients. It was all the little things I enjoyed the most, but mainly my ability to function in society and help those who still could not help themselves.

I was tasked with visiting patients in their homes to assist them with tasks they were no longer able to do alone. I was responsible for making sure they took a shower, dressed, and had food to eat. I would also perform medical care, which involved testing their glucose levels, helping them with their vitals, and cleaning their wounds where required. The patients often had questions or concerns, and it was my role to report these to the nurse in charge of their care. My connection with them was so genuine – I knew how it felt to be isolated and immobile.

Every day felt like it was worth living. Pain medication was no longer holding me down, and my daily purpose was clear - to look after my family, help my patients, and be active wherever I could be. Rob was so much more relaxed, my mother was able to get on with her life back in Florida, and I could ferry my boys around and cook for my family once again. The power of my decision to apply for that job was overwhelming; just look at the results. It all happened when I started believing in myself again. I made a mindful decision that opened so many doors. Only I could decide when to change, but the support I received from my family was invaluable in helping me to take those steps.

If you find yourself feeling concerned for someone in a similar situation, do not give up on them. It may not seem like they are listening to you, but kind, motivating words do get absorbed and do make a difference.

As the months passed, I was looking forward to the rest of my life.

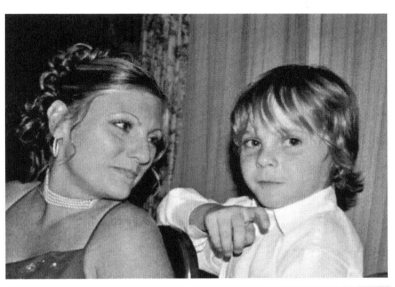

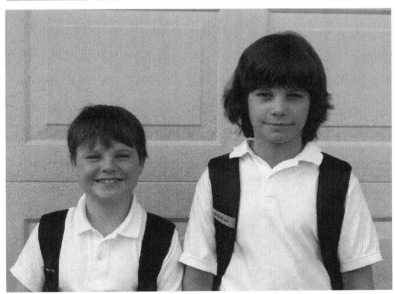

CHAPTER 8

Corruption

My days were busy, but it felt so rewarding to be helping the less able. I had one patient who suffered from Dementia and was very unstable. I visited his house daily and always tried to leave him with a smile. Taking time out of my day to talk to him was important to me.

One morning, I visited him after dropping my boys off at school. His daughter was there, and he was much happier than his usual self. The showering process was never straightforward. Despite repeatedly advising his family to install a shower bench, they insisted on using a lawn chair instead. I reported this to my office, in my notes, on numerous occasions, but I was always told to *"make do with what they have."* His daughter volunteered to help me move him from his bed to his wheelchair, and from there, we took him directly to the shower room. He kept trying to stand up and walk, but he was not physically strong enough to carry his own body weight. I had a firm hold on him until we reached the shower and then helped him into the lawn chair. As I began to wash him, I was talking to him in a desperate attempt to keep his mind occupied, but he was adamant about standing up. Then, out of nowhere, he launched himself out of the lawn chair and slipped.

I reacted fast to catch all 180lbs of him.
Thankfully, he did not suffer any damage.

Unfortunately for me, when I reacted suddenly to prevent him from falling, I felt a 'POP' in my lower spine, followed by a burning sensation in my back. Frightened, worried, and distraught, I had to get him out of the shower and back into his wheelchair - as quickly as possible.

Panic was setting in, but I was determined to complete my tasks calmly and professionally, and without causing a scene. I called for his daughter to come and help me. She rushed over, and together we dressed him and helped him back into bed. I did what I needed to do, left the house, and went straight to my car. I instinctively knew that something was wrong. Has a screw popped in my lower spine? Has a rod slipped out of place? All the questions, all at once. I sat in my car, took a few deep breaths, and focused intently on what to do next.

My intuition led me directly to the office to speak to my supervisor. I answered all her questions and told her everything as we filled out the necessary paperwork for 'getting injured on the job.' She then informed me to visit the Human Resources doctor's office right away. I drove there slowly feeling scared and confused by what had just happened. I did not want to know what the doctor had to say, and certainly not what this meant for my future.

An overwhelming sense of pessimism was taking over my entire body and mind. It was a darker version of myself, and there was nothing I could do to stop her. The pain was getting worse by the second. I felt physically sick as I pulled up outside the Medical Center. Was I about to lose this career I had built for myself?

I often think about the challenges of life and how everything can change in the blink of an eye. Life changed for me when I broke my back, but I believed I would recover. I spoke to the doctor and explained my situation. He felt the muscles in my back, had me move into different positions, and told me they had *"locked up."* He ordered an x-ray immediately. I did not know exactly what to expect, but I knew the results were not going to be good.

"Michelle, it seems nothing too serious has happened. All your hardware is intact, but you have pulled a muscle in your lower back. You need to rest and allow four weeks to heal." he said bluntly.

They told me that I would still get paid, but under no circumstances was I allowed to work. How could this be happening to me? No work for four weeks? He prescribed a mixture of muscle relaxers and pain relief meds to help me manage the pain. Reluctantly, I accepted the prescriptions and told him I looked forward to the day I could return to work. Strangely, as I walked out of his office, I knew I wasn't going back.

All I wanted to do was work and function normally - two things I used to take for granted. A couple of weeks into my leave, I received a call from Human Resources. They were calling to let me know that a Care Manager was being assigned to my case. Having worked in the medical field, I knew the real motive behind 'Care' Managers. Although we are led to believe that they are there to ensure we receive 'proper care', the truth is quite different. A Care Manager is a nurse that goes with you to all your medical appointments to ensure you are not 'milking the system'. Their primary goal is to see you go back to work as soon as possible because the employer is responsible for paying your medical bills and wages. Of course, they will do everything in their power not to pay.

I scheduled an appointment with my neurosurgeon, to find out if the hardware in my lower back was still intact. He was the doctor I trusted in the first place to insert the screws and rods during the first Spinal Fusion surgery, and I wanted a piece of his mind. He ordered an MRI scan before the appointment, meaning we would have the results to discuss during the meeting.

My Care Manager met us at his office on the day of the appointment. Following an exam, my neurosurgeon confirmed that the injury was caused by severely pulled muscles and that the disc at L5-S1 was mildly herniated, causing the nerve pain to travel down my right leg. He prescribed more muscle relaxers and pain medication and informed the Care Manager that I needed twelve weeks to recover, not four.

My employers were not satisfied with that conclusion and insisted I see one of 'their' neurosurgeons instead. Of course, I was always open to a second opinion and welcomed the idea of having a fresh set of eyes review my test results. Part of me believed they were doing this as part of a genuine attempt to help me get back to work, but I could not have been more wrong. As I arrived at the meeting with one of 'their' neurosurgeons, I handed over my x-rays and MRI films. His response was not what I had expected.

"Your back is fine, Michelle. You can return to work now," he said.

What did this mean? My neurosurgeon, who I trusted, told me I needed twelve weeks to heal. Now, I had 'their' neurosurgeon telling me that everything was fine and that I should return to work immediately. What about the herniated disc, and constant pain? He reassured me that my back was fine, and that all hardware was intact. As he spoke to me, he was signing the release papers that permitted me to return to work, and before I had a chance to ask any questions, he had left the room.

Something did not feel right, and as I gathered my belongings and left the building, the conversation kept replaying in my head. I was upset and felt mistreated by someone who was supposed to care about the health and well-being of others. It felt as if a line of hot burning acid was constantly running down my leg and into my foot. I could not sleep at night, and was reliant, once again, on pharmaceutical drugs. How could I work without sleep and on high doses of medication? None of it made any sense at all.

A couple of days later, I received a certified letter from my employer. The letter stated I had three days to return to work or I would get fired.

I called her right away to find out what was going on. Staying calm proved to be difficult as I swallowed my tears in between words. I took a deep breath and explained that I was physically unable to return to work due to the intense pain I was suffering. I reminded her that my neurosurgeon had advised for twelve weeks to heal and that I had not yet been signed off as 'fit for work.' She did not say much, and the conversation ended. Four days later, I received another certified letter. This letter stated that my employment had been terminated.

How could they tell me that my back was 'fine,' and I should return to work immediately? The x-rays clearly showed a herniated disc. I decided to research the doctor's name online to find out more about him. It did not take me long to find a mountain of bad reviews written by previous patients. He was not only doing this to me but getting paid by this large and reputable healthcare company to sign release papers for injured staff to return to work - regardless of their physical condition! With his approval, the employer can avoid paying medical bills and wages for employees who get injured on the job. I could not believe some of the stuff I was reading.

My faith in humanity was a challenge to uphold. Rob convinced me that what they were doing was illegal and said that due to the fact I was under doctor's care with strict orders 'not to return to work,' they could not legally fire me.

He insisted we hire a lawyer.

I agreed, and we were recommended a lawyer by Rob's boss. Rob made the first call, and the feedback was positive. The lawyer told him that we had a strong case and booked an appointment for us to discuss everything in more detail.

CHAPTER 9

The Great Recession

He agreed to represent me. This lawyer had experience in dealing with these types of cases and was already familiar with the doctor we were acting against. We signed the paperwork, and the case was filed. It felt good to be fighting back with some solid support for once. I was on track to sue the big healthcare company that fired me illegally. It only took two court appearances from my attorney before they came back with a settlement offer. I accepted the offer at $12,500.00 and the case was closed.

Rob had come to the rescue again and given me the strength I needed to keep fighting. I felt empowered by the fact that I had exercised my right to justice and won! I was left with $7,500.00 after the legal fees were deducted, and grateful for every penny. We used that money to pay off accumulating debt, our past-due mortgage payments, and took a weekend vacation with the boys to a waterpark. It was great to be doing something as a family and to see them all so happy. For me, it was a different experience as I walked through the waterpark with pain meds flowing through my bloodstream. It was difficult for anyone to understand how much energy I needed to generate to complete the simplest of tasks. Nevertheless, I felt we had achieved a positive step in the right direction and refused to let my pain ruin this enjoyable weekend away.

As time went on, the pain got worse.

I was back to being unemployed, in constant pain, and only doing the bare minimum as a wife and mom. My doctor suggested I see a pain management doctor for different medications and to administer spinal steroid injections to further ease the pain. I found a local pain doctor online, and after reading his stellar reviews on the internet, made an appointment to meet him. He immediately increased my Norco prescription from 7.5mg to 10mg, every 4 hours, added Gabapentin at 750mg, every 6 hours, and more muscle relaxers.   My quality of life was disintegrating, and I was fast becoming dependent on this legal yet lethal concoction of pain medications. But this time was quite different from the last. The saying, **'you can't help someone who does not want to be helped'** is, absolutely true. I did not want help. I did not want to know. The magic stuff was easing the pain, and that is how I felt safe.

I believed the meds were keeping me alive.

As a steady supply of drugs blanketed my days, I was viciously thrust back into a life of dark addiction. By 2009, The Great Recession had arrived, and we were secretly living through incredibly challenging times. We had mounting medical bills exceeding $130,000.00, hockey fees for both boys, equipment fees, tournament fees, and more. We were behind on our mortgage payments, again, and our phones would not stop ringing. Banks and creditors were always calling for money, and we had our everyday living costs to consider too. On the other hand, we felt lucky to still have our family home, and whatever income Rob got from unemployment was spent mainly on the boys so that they could continue living a normal life. Behind the scenes, our debt continued to rise out of control, and my addiction to pharmaceutical drugs was getting worse. When I felt pain, I popped a pain pill. When I felt sad, I popped a pain pill. When I felt confused, I popped a pain pill; I was no longer numbing just the physical pain.

I attended monthly appointments with the pain doctor, and every month he increased my dosage. Once I had reached the maximum dosage of one pain medicine, he would prescribe something much stronger. It was not long before I had a prescription for 240 Dilaudid pills for one month. These were 4mg pills that numbed me as no other medicine did. In my mind, the Dilaudid pills launched me into another dimension entirely. I had no idea what normality was anymore and did not wish to find out. Being numb was all that mattered to me.

As the Great Recession took its toll on society, my family became yet another statistic among the many facing struggle and turmoil. Was I thriving to be the best wife and mother I could be to protect my family? No, by no means was I. My days were spent, mostly in bed, with the housework piling up around me. My boys were always running around playing, but I had no energy to give them. It reached a point where they had to eat cereal for dinner, most nights. I was failing miserably at being a mom and was not the wife I had vowed to be, all those years before. Mentally, I had escaped so far and was not thinking about what effect my behavior was having on my family.

I could not even change the bed sheets for my children, and I was still choosing drugs over motherhood.

Opioid pain relievers were declared as '**not addictive**' in medical communities, throughout the United States, during the late 1990s. Consequently, healthcare providers became much more lenient with their prescription dosages and issued more drugs more often. It was only later revealed that these medications could be '**highly addictive**,' and in 2017, a public health emergency was declared. The U.S. Opioid Epidemic was born, and while some victims still seek rehabilitation, others fast turned to illegal drugs, overdose, and suicide. The U.S. Opioid Epidemic continues to create communities of 'illegal' and 'legal' drug users. The problem is that even legal drugs are not safe to use. There was barely any difference in my behavior from that of a heroin user. Whether opioids are categorized into legally manufactured medications or illicit narcotics, the effects can still be the same. I was of no sane mind under the influence of these legal drugs.

Rob soon found work at a local car dealership, working exceptionally long hours. This should have given me motivation and a reason to feel safer and happier, but I still could not change. Walking my pup or preparing a tasty homemade meal was still not on my list of things to do each day.

My boys never complained about my spiritual absence and always kept themselves occupied by playing video games or playing outside. It was obvious to me that my husband was suffering, but what could he do? I was not listening to anything he told me. I had neglected my family, and still live with guilt every single day for that. As far as I was concerned, the only things I had to achieve each day were taking my meds and getting the boys to and from school. Driving was not an easy task for me and most definitely not the safest option for my beloved children. The rest of my time was spent, in bed, numb.

I have no recollection of Christmas 2009.

CHAPTER 10
Eviction

Anyone suffering from addiction and depression will most likely know what it feels like to hit rock bottom. Imagine waking up every single day what it feels like to hit rock bottom. Imagine waking up every single day wishing you had not. Imagine feeling that your family would be better off without you and that by ending your life, you would be doing them a favor. Non-sufferers often describe suicide as a selfish act, but, when you live without purpose, and in constant pain, it feels like a decision that would benefit the ones you love. Despite receiving guidance from a legitimate medical provider, I had become addicted, like every other drug addict out there.

There was no way out, as far as my eye could see, and the walls were caving in on me, more and more. The dark circles under my eyes were a clear sign of my irregular sleeping patterns, and my lack of energy was something everyone had gotten used to. I could not fall asleep before 2 or 3 am, and every day, my alarm would sound at 5:30 am, just in time for the school run. I would wake up feeling tired and drowsy from the medicine, still in my system from the night before. Regardless, I managed the school run successfully most days. It is, however, fair to say that if the boys did not want to go to school, I did not try to persuade them otherwise. I simply agreed so that I did not have to get in the car and drive them. This made me the *"best mom ever"* in their eyes, but I knew I was being a terrible mother. I convinced myself that my condition was only temporary and that eventually, I would get better, and things would go back to how they were before the accident. If I had not committed myself to do the school runs, I doubt I would have ever left the house. Adopting a positive mindset was becoming harder to achieve as the months passed by. The pain was still getting worse.

In early 2010, my sister revealed that she was pregnant with her first child. As you can imagine, this was such an exciting time for our family! It had been quite a few years since we had had a new life born into our immediate family, and as she lived just a few doors down, I knew I was going to be a big part of this baby's life.

My husband was back in employment working for a local car dealership, and my boys were happy, healthy, and actively involved with their hockey teams. I had so many reasons to be thankful and feel hopeful about our future, but I could not do it. I could not pull myself out of my rut. The lethal combination of pain meds and depression was gripping me tightly and refusing to let me go! I felt trapped with no way of escaping.

Then, something horrific happened.

I was getting the boys ready for school one morning, and as usual, I had not managed to sleep well due to pain. I also felt drowsy and tired from the pain meds I had taken before going to bed. I pushed my feelings to the side and carried myself through the motions of getting my boys to school.

We got in the car to begin our journey, and as we were driving along, I suddenly heard Kyle scream *"MOM!"* at the top of his lungs. I slammed on the brakes and only just escaped rear-ending the stopped car in front – by an inch! Overwhelmed by feelings of guilt and concern for my boys and myself, I tried to cover up what had just happened. I immediately said, *"Mommy was just distracted, looking out the window,"* apologized for my carelessness, and hoped that they would forgive me. Kane was too young to understand the severity of my deterioration, but Kyle could see straight through me. He knew exactly what was going on. I was foolish to ever think that he couldn't.

That experience served as a shocking wake-up call for me. I had nodded off at the wheel and was milliseconds away from putting my boy's lives at risk, the other driver's, and my own. The thought of even putting myself in a position where I allowed such a thing to happen, angers me to this day. I could have caused the death of my children as a direct result of being addicted to opioids. I did not know how to stop abusing pain medication, but for the first time in a long time, I wanted to find out.

I wanted to stop but was afraid of the pain without it.

Stuck between a rock and a hard place, I decided to slow down my intake by stretching out the time in between doses. I hoped this would be the start to something better, but my efforts to slow down only lasted a few months. I may have seemed a little less absent, but I was still in a lot of pain and spent most of my days in bed. Reducing my dosage was not only a mental challenge but also a reminder of how much I was numbing the physical pain in the first place.   Pain serves as a way for our bodies to communicate with us and alert us to the fact that something may be wrong. Wiping out those signs by numbing them, and pretending they do not exist, is not the way forward if you want to heal.

I know that now.

We had fallen so far behind on our mortgage payments, and letters marked in red with 'Confidential' or 'Urgent' appeared daily in our mailbox. My solution to this problem was to keep ignoring them and continue living with my head in the clouds. This made life harder for Rob, as I had become self-centered. I was still dependent on the drugs. I was no longer living my life but existing in everyone else's. I never used to think about how my sons perceived me when I was under the influence of pain medication; I believed they could not tell the difference. I had convinced myself that saying *"I love you,"* and squeezing a smile in their presence was good enough to make me a good mom, but my perception of reality was warped, and, although aware, I didn't know what to do to help myself. I wanted to stop, but the only thing I still fought for was my next prescription. Letters from debt collectors continued to arrive in our mailbox, and our phones would not stop ringing. In October, we received a knock on the door from the local Sheriff.

He had come to deliver our Eviction Notice.

It was a devastating time for all of us as we were about to lose the last thing we had left and valued so much: **our family home.** The foundation we laid to raise our family, the structure we designed, built, and called home for seventeen years was about to be taken from our lives forever. Worse than that, there was absolutely nothing we could do about it. My nightmare was becoming a reality, and I have never felt as useless as I did then. It was the only home my boys ever knew, and making memories there was about to end. Rob needed me to get my act together. I had to be there for him like he is always there for me! We were about to become homeless in just a few months if we did not take evasive action.

Forcing myself to reengage with my senses, I built the courage to address the inevitable. Rob and I had to tell the boys we were going to be moving out of our home. We discussed the best time to tell them, how to do it, and how to make it easy for them to accept. We decided to view it as a learning curve instead of bad news and went with the approach that 'change is good.' I guess we were also trying to convince ourselves that it could be a positive transition. My boys are sharp cookies and were smart enough to see what was happening; there was no way of hiding the torture we were going through.

Every day, my heart broke for my husband who ruthlessly blamed himself. He felt so guilty for not being able to save our home. At the same time, I blamed myself, thinking that if I had not broken my back, none of this would have happened. I could have continued working and not created so much medical debt. If only I had avoided those stairs that day, if only I had been more careful. If only.

We were given two months to prepare and had to be out of our home by January 2011.

CHAPTER 11
Misunderstandings

Although I clutch onto my belief that everything happens for a reason, I could not find the reason for why all of this was happening to me. November the 1st, 2010; I remember it clearly. My sister gave birth to a healthy and beautiful baby girl. They called her Fiona Grace, and just like that, we were blessed with a new addition to our family. We all love children and were so excited for my sister and her husband. Luckily, they only lived a few doors down, so my boys were able to visit their newborn cousin regularly, and I was able to show my support too. I was devastated by the fact we would soon be evicted from our family home and forced to move elsewhere. Nevertheless, a new and innocent bundle of energy named Fiona was welcomed into a loving family, bringing us all that little bit closer.

My grandparents had always played a significant role in my upbringing, and my respect for them will always be strong. They went through a lot to support me as a child, and despite my grandmother's own personal health issues and back problems, she never gave up. My fondest childhood memories are the times spent with my grandparents.

I have always found it interesting how our minds decide on which memories to keep. I remember sitting in their living room, eating cheese and butter sandwiches on Roman Meal bread, while grandma stood ironing sheets and underwear! She always did the ironing while watching the soap opera, As the World Turns, and would sing during her long cooking sessions in the kitchen. I spent so much time with my grandmother because we only lived nine doors down. Later in life, we moved to an apartment in Chicago, and that was directly above them.

Both my grandparents would babysit me while my mom was in Beauty School and while my dad worked long shifts as a Chicago Police Officer. They also owned a gorgeous country cottage in Wisconsin and would visit there almost every weekend during the summer months. Whenever they mentioned the cottage, I would get so excited, and I remember begging to go with them because I just loved it there! They never refused me and always let me tag along.

For me, it was like having extra sets of parents taking care of me. I adored being with them, but I also remember grandpa telling me, *"Grandma is in bed,"* quite often. As a child, you do not think about why things are the way they are and accept what you are being told as the truth. I never questioned why she was in bed and continued spending time with her as if nothing were different. I would still visit her and sit at her bedside singing Church songs I had learned in Catholic School. I played with her jewelry, pranced around her bedroom, and hid in her closet, playing with dresses and shoes. It was only as I grew older that I learned she had back problems and suffered severe chronic pain. As a child, I did not understand what she was going through, but I do have memories of her lying in bed, wearing a hard plastic brace, and looking very tired.

Despite the hardships she faced, my grandmother always remained elegant. No matter how bad things got, she always dressed up. I do not recall ever seeing her without earrings on, a watch on, and hair made up. She was a proud and beautiful woman who loved me as if I were her daughter. I continued to visit them regularly as I grew older, and even after they moved permanently to their cottage in Wisconsin, I always found time to drive over and see them. My adamance to never lose our connection was strong, and no matter how my grandmother felt, she never turned down a visit. I can still hear her voice now, saying, *"Yes, come on over, Michelle."* It was not unusual for her to go to bed halfway through our visit, but we didn't mind. My grandfather and I used that time to have a good catch-up, discuss life, and make supper, ready for when she woke up again.

My boys also loved it there. We have so many comforting memories of the two of them playing for hours in the garden and riding their bikes up and down the rocky roads, again and again. You could always hear them laughing as they chased frogs along the creek, and one of their favorite pastimes was playing with cars and trucks among the rocks, in the forest nearby. It filled me with so much happiness to see them so content. That regular dose of fresh air and nature was always a blessing for all of us.

As the years passed by, her physical condition continued to deteriorate. As her back pain worsened, it became clear that she was struggling to cope. Watching her try and hide her pain was sad yet inspiring at the same time. The last thing she wanted to do was burden anyone with her pain. It crossed my mind a few times that she may be overmedicating on pain medicine, but I did not understand the severity of that until later in life. She was my backbone throughout all my surgeries, and despite her suffering, she still found the energy to call me regularly. My grandmother understood me more than anyone else I knew and always encouraged me to fight harder. Constant reminders to be confident and stay strong for my husband and sons, have stayed with me to this day. I do not know where I would be without her ongoing support and unconditional love.

Sadly, around 2010, my grandmother was becoming increasingly forgetful and more frustrated as a result. She would get angry over the smallest of things and was often snippy on the phone to me. Her words would sting me at first, but I knew that she was not an angry woman and would never, under normal circumstances, ever talk to me like that. We believe that dementia had started setting in, and as time went on, her condition worsened. I remember times when she even struggled to recognize my grandfather.

When Fiona was born, on November the 1st, 2010, my mom had traveled from Florida to meet her first granddaughter and to be there to help with my sisters' recovery. She had also scheduled a knee surgery for the day after Fiona's birth. My mom and I visited my sister in the hospital where we met Fiona for the first time. She was such a beautiful baby, and my sister was in good spirits. The following morning, we were up at 5am going back to the hospital for mom's knee surgery. Not forgetting I had a fair few problems in the pipeline and was only weeks away from losing our family home, I still did everything in my power to be there and support my mom and sister as best I could. It was important to me that I could be there for them as they were for me throughout everything. As we got in the car to head home after mom's surgery, my cell phone rang.

It was my grandmother, and she was furious! Never, in 41 years, had I heard so much anger in her voice. *"Did you not think to call me when your sister had her baby?"* she yelled. It was so out of character for her that I cannot describe in words how this affected me; I was thrown by her tone. Reminding myself about her condition, I calmly explained that I had planned to call her a little later in the day. I told her how busy we had been, but she did not care at all. She was mad at me. I was stunned by what she was saying and had mixed feelings about how I should respond. I was doing my best to take care of mom, be on-call for my sister, husband, and sons, when all my body needed to do was rest. Then, in a moment of pure rage, my compassion neglected me, and I unleashed my anger on her, my beloved grandmother. I shouted back at her and told her in one breath what I was going through, how I was losing my home, and how I was just trying to take care of my sister and mom. I was angry that she had called me and screamed at me with such venom in her tone. Who was that person talking to me in such a way? I reminded her that my dad had already called her about the birth and proceeded to call her 'ridiculous' for wanting to hear it from me too.

What was I thinking?

Her response killed me. *"Michelle is your mother with you?"* she asked. *"Yes, I told you, I am driving her home from the hospital,"* I responded

68

abruptly. *"It figures, you have an audience!"* she said. I immediately hung up on her. I did not say a word and did not say goodbye. She had <u>never</u> spoken to me like that before. In a moment where I should have shown great understanding and empathy, my mind crumbled and tears streamed down my face. For days, I felt broken. She did not call me back; I did not call her back. This regret will stay with me for the rest of my life.

Two days later, she fell ill and was rushed to the hospital. As soon as I received the news, I dropped what I was doing and went to see her at once. My grandfather was there. I will never forget the way he glared at me as I entered the room. He looked disgusted with me. Shivers traveled through my spine as I saw my grandmother lay unconscious on the bed. I felt physically sick and have never felt so scared in my life. I walked over to the bed, but she was so heavily sedated that I will never know if she was even aware of my presence. I held her hand and apologized repeatedly. We had never fought before; she had never even yelled at me once! This could not be real. Why could I not wake up from this nightmare? I begged her to respond to me, but she never did. Was I about to lose one of the most important and loving people in my life? These were the people that loved me as their daughter. What was happening? There was nothing I could do to put things right.

My beloved grandmother was taken by angels on November 11th, 2010, with my grandfather at her bedside.

I did not see my grandfather again until the day of her wake. I spent a lot of time trying to focus and prepare myself mentally for the event, but nothing could have prepared me for what I saw upon arriving at the funeral home. I saw her body, completely lifeless. I was inconsolable, broken. My role model left this world, with us being on the worst of terms. My dear grandmother never got to see me again, or hear me say, *"I am sorry."* I missed my only chance to make amends, and she died during a fight with me that should never have taken place. I will never get the chance to fix what I broke. My grandfather held my hand throughout most of the wake.

After the service, he walked with me to the casket. He spoke in a calm voice and said something to my grandmother that I will hold with me forever.

"Michelle was here for you. Our daughter was here," he whispered.

ALWAYS REMEMBERING MARY CARIOSCIA
SEPTEMBER 27TH 1925 – NOVEMBER 11TH 2010

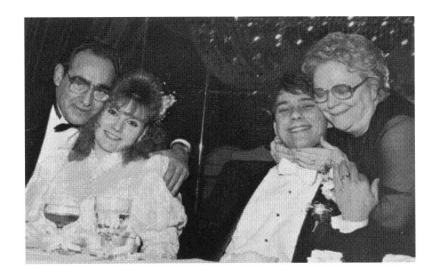

CHAPTER 12

Guilt

Living with guilt presented a whole new level of emotion I had not experienced before. There was not enough Norco in the entire world to ease that pain. Every day, I woke up with a heavy heart and reached for the Norco. Mentally, things seemed to get better after my morning fix, which helped to numb the guilt and fear of losing our family home.

We were just weeks away from being evicted and still had no action plan or place to go. By December of 2010, my husband and I were left with no choice but to join forces and find a solution. We discussed housing options, but funds were so limited, and we had pets to consider too. We were both petrified about our future, our boys, and how the eviction might affect their schooling arrangements. Were they going to be forced away from their childhood friends into a new school and area? How would they settle in? What if they didn't? How would they continue attending their hockey clubs? Would we be able to visit my sister and little Fiona? The questions kept repeating through my mind.

Each day, Rob searched for houses to rent in our neighborhood and tried to show me the listings of suitable properties available. I knew that we had zero chance of securing a rental because we had defaulted on our mortgage, and our credit was so bad! Rob kept up the pace and remained optimistic, but I knew that nobody would rent to us and did not feel the need to waste my time looking. Then, one morning, Rob walks into the room with a huge grin on his face, looking very excited. *"Get in the car, Michelle. I have found a house for us!"* he said confidently. I immediately feared that he was getting his hopes up too much. I was in such a negative state of mind that I *could* not and *would* not get excited with him. The house was in the next neighborhood, and an appointment had been made with the realtor who had agreed to meet us there. It all seemed a bit too good to be true.

The house was more than just beautiful.

The bedrooms were large and spacious for the boys, and the master bedroom had a master ensuite bathroom! The kitchen was neatly tiled with beautiful ceramic tiles throughout, and there was even a huge fenced-in yard for my Little Boo. Part of me was overwhelmed by its perfection, but of course, the other part of me was still depressed because I did not believe we stood half a chance of securing this house for a new home. Rob asked all the necessary questions and conversed with the realtor in detail. She explained that a Pastor owned the house and had recently moved out of town to work at another church. She seemed pretty confident that if we told the Pastor our story, he would give us a chance. All I had to do was write a letter detailing everything that had happened to us, and how we desperately needed this opportunity to start our lives over. We went home, wrote the letter, sent it off, and waited in anticipation for the Pastor's response. Two days passed. I still had my doubts, but Rob was hopeful. Then, three days later, he received a call from the realtor. She informed him that Pastor Mark's response was positive and talked about his belief that everyone deserves a second chance.

Pastor Mark had agreed to rent us his house!

We could not believe our luck! We were so overwhelmed and cried tears of joy. I cannot describe how proud I was (and still am) of my husband for keeping up the bravery and powering through like a true soldier. He stayed strong when I failed to, and, as a result, a beautiful new home was waiting for us in the next neighborhood! Everything was so surreal. We were going to be okay. The boys could continue at the same school, keep the same friends, and attend their hockey club as they had done for so many years. We could still visit my sister and little Fiona, and the heavy grey cloud was finally floating away from above our heads. My mindset shifted as the excitement increased. We made the most of each day by sharing our excellent news with the boys. If we got excited, they got excited, and Boo got excited too! Christmas was just a couple of weeks away, and so was eviction day.

I have clear memories of our Christmas tree, sitting pretty, next to a pile of boxes that were packed and stacked with items from our living room. I was still overmedicated but felt happy to see my husband and sons smiling again. Sadly, I could not stop thinking about how my grandmother was no longer with us, and nothing could help me unload the guilt I lived with every day. I took Norco with my coffee, every morning before the boys even woke up, and despite being our very last Christmas in our family home, I did absolutely nothing to make it a memorable one. After all my husband had done for us, it was the least I could have done.

Christmas 2010 was far from a Christmas to remember.
We decided to move into our new home on the 2nd of January 2011, at the start of a fresh new year. Rob and I felt it would be better to leave on our terms instead of being forced out. Our family helped so much with the move, and we still feel blessed to this day for all the hard work they invested. A large weight was immediately lifted from our shoulders. We all settled in brilliantly.

In February of 2011, my husband was offered a respectable job position out of state in Wisconsin. He accepted, and our financial situation also began to improve. Our future was looking brighter than it had done for a long time. I had every reason to be happy, and every bit of support I needed to get myself back on the straight and narrow. However, my priorities still did not change. Nothing mattered to me anymore. If I could get up in the morning, take my meds, and get the boys to and from school, I was doing my part as far as I was concerned. Most of my days and nights were still spent in bed, numb.

I knew I needed to stop, but I was addicted.

Any excuse I could think of to keep taking the meds was a good excuse. What kind of wife and mother had I become? If I did not act fast, I was going to kill myself or someone close to me. I spent quite a few months battling with my thoughts. It was not easy, but I carried on telling myself that I no longer wanted to live like a zombie and that if I wanted to get my life back, it was up to me. Every time I looked at my husband and sons, I built up more guilt and started feeling repulsed at myself for not being stronger. I could not even be an aunt to my little niece, Fiona.

It was time to get my head out of my backside and do something about it. It took a while for me to realize that if I did not do something different, nothing would change. I did not stop using pain medicine straight away because I did not know how to manage the pain without it. I needed professional guidance to get me back into the real world, but for me to achieve that successfully, I had to want the help and take steps to find it myself.

It was as if someone else had taken over my being, and was guiding me out of the rut I was in. Was it my grandmother? I like to think it was. I always think about how my mind changed so suddenly. It was a strange sensation to experience after being stuck for so long, but I wanted it so bad that I did not waste a second. I started researching online to source recommended Rehabilitation Centers in the area and found a place in downtown Chicago, which suited my criteria perfectly.

I registered to begin Rehab in July of 2011.

CHAPTER 13

Transition

The night before I was due to start Rehab remains a prominent memory in my mind. I remember lying in bed with millions of thoughts and questions racing through my head at lightning speed. Why did all of this happen to me? How have I become this person? Why has my life crumbled like this? What kind of mother am I? How have I become such a useless wife? Where are my friends? Why are my family members turning against me? I remember finding out they had been talking negatively about me, which led to more feelings of confusion and isolation. I had known for a long time that Rehab was the best decision for me, but I was so scared. How will I manage the pain without medication? How will I handle the harsh effects of withdrawal? How will I find the courage to speak openly with strangers about my story? Won't they judge me? Who will sit with me at lunch? Do we get lunch?

I was beginning to feel nauseous.

The next morning was the one we had all been waiting for. I had spent months thinking about what it was going to be like, whether I was going to be able to cope, and struggled to understand how they were going to help me manage the pain without the meds. It is so hard to comprehend until you get there and listen to what they have to say. I knew it was a two-hour journey there and back, but I was determined to do this and put a stop to all our suffering. On the first day, my husband drove me to the train station. I was trembling uncontrollably and doubted myself and my ability to complete the course. Traveling alone was also something I had been dreading, but it had to be done. I was terrified, to begin with, but somehow, I knew it was the right decision. ***"You've got this Michelle!"*** Rob said. **"Go!"**

and I did. I reminded myself repeatedly that I was doing the right thing and put one foot in front of the other until I reached the door of the Rehabilitation Institute of Chicago (RIC). As I opened the door, I knew I was opening the door to a new life. My husband and boys deserved this just as much as I needed it.

The RIC describes itself as the **'first-ever translational research hospital where clinicians, scientists, innovators, and technologists work together in the same space, applying research in real time to physical medicine and rehabilitation.'** I was welcomed into a hygienic, friendly, and organized space where skilled nurses were always available to help. It was fully equipped with all the latest technology and designed to ensure a calm and healthy healing environment. I had procrastinated for so long but was surprised to discover that I felt safe there.

We were placed into small intimate groups of six people. Despite our major life differences, we were all on a similar journey and were able to understand one another without much effort. My small group in Rehab connected well together, and I was shocked to find that these were people just like me. Each one of them had been prescribed pain medication for an injury or medical condition, and each one of them had nearly lost their life to medication addiction. These were not homeless people living on the street or in dark corners across the city; these were mothers, fathers, businessmen, and women. In our group, we also had a lawyer and a firefighter.

These were normal, hard-working people that, like me, nearly had their lives destroyed by profit-driven doctors and so-called medical experts.

We had been gifted each other and were handed the tools we needed to heal. We all had one thing in common; to get off the pharmaceutical drugs and reconnect with ourselves. It felt liberating. They showed great support when I spoke about my pain, my circumstances, and my emotions. They wanted to know the details as I wanted to know theirs. For the first time in a long time, I no longer felt unwanted. It was extremely comforting, knowing that you could speak openly and freely without feeling like a burden. These people really got me!

Many have asked me what a typical day at Rehab is like.

The first and most important thing we learned was to understand the **difference between physical and emotional pain**. Our mission was to embrace a new, spiritual journey, find our inner calm, and learn how to live without the drugs. Each day we were tasked with a different schedule consisting of five hours of hard work. A typical day started in a Nursing Class, where we learned about pain, nutrition, and the effects of pain medication on the body. We were also taught about stress levels and how they negatively impact our physical being and wellness.

Then, we would attend a Psychology Class with alternating days of group and individual therapy, usually followed by the Occupational Therapy Group. This was where we were taught about basic body mechanics, relating to how to sit, stand, and reach properly while coping with our diagnosed medical conditions.

After, we would attend the Biofeedback Group, where we learned about the Mind-Body connection and how to channel your focus onto something other than your pain. I was skeptical about this class, to begin with, and admittedly gave the instructor a hard time with my inquisitive and persistent questioning. It turned out to be one of the most effective classes that helped me to control my pain. The fine line between Pain Management and Medication Addiction was becoming clear to me.

I had become so dependent on the drugs that I was no longer medicating just my physical pain.

I felt a shift in my awareness as I came true to myself. Attending Rehab awakened me from a dark place where there was no light at the end of the tunnel. How did I not know about nutrition and natural self-healing before becoming a pain med junkie? How is this not common knowledge for everyone? Is this a flaw in our education system or a personal naivety? I promised myself to stop living in denial; I had been living a lie for far too long and was on a mission to complete Rehab for me and my family.

The last class of every day was Physical Training, which included yoga, meditation, stretching, and Feldenkrais. Feldenkrais was the most popular method and became my favorite class of all. It was through Feldenkrais that I finally learned how to **'shift my pain.'**

The Feldenkrais Method changed my life.

Dr. Moshe Feldenkrais was a Ukrainian Israeli engineer, physicist, and founder of the **Feldenkrais Method**. His revolutionary approach to healing has changed the lives of millions worldwide, including mine. I was guided through a series of **awareness-throughmovement** classes that focused on slow exercise routines designed to achieve powerful effects on flexibility, strength, balance, and holistic integration of the Body and Mind. I was shown how to use gentle, mindful movements, which helped me to understand the connection between my brain and physical body, in ways I never thought possible; my physical and mental capacity was improving! One of the most unique and inspiring aspects of this somatic education is that the techniques are designed to help you in everyday life. The movements tie directly into your day-to-day functional activities, including keeping a good posture, sitting, walking, lifting objects, and general stretching routines. Instead of feeling crippled and useless, I was slowly learning to use what I had to help me feel better.

By attending the regular classes, the painful muscular tension that had had me crippled for so long began to release and reorganize. I went for many years without thinking pragmatically about my circumstances. It took professional psychologists to unravel my confusion and help me think logically. Everything made sense once I had become clear-headed enough to realize the facts.

- How can we improve brain function if we do not understand it?
- How can we master efficient movement if we do not learn the connection between Body and Mind?
- How can we heal fast if we do not know what is wrong?
- How can we improve our sense of being when we are too numb to feel anything at all?

We went on to learn about Chakra Healing Energy and how to use it in controlling our consciousness. Our chakras act as a vortex for the constant energy flow into and out of our bodies and help regulate our body's processes, including organ function, immune system, and emotions. Everything in our Universe radiates energy, and that includes each individual cell in our bodies. I was aware of Chakra Healing before I attended Rehab, but I had no real understanding of its importance in our lives. Interacting with various physiological and neurological systems, our chakras offer different benefits depending on where they are located in the body.

We each have hundreds of chakras, but only seven main chakras are typically dealt with for healing and cleansing purposes. They begin at the bottom of the spine and run along your spinal cord to the very highest point at the crown of your head. It makes sense that when our chakras stop functioning or become blocked, the energy flow fizzles out, and so do we. We were taught how to cleanse our chakras frequently to reach a place of balance between Spirit, Body, and Earth.

From experience, I would say that self-awareness is the key to self healing. The most challenging times we face are there to teach us, how to react, how to cope, and how to heal. I endured years of excruciating pain before I learned about Neuromuscular Reprogramming.

In hindsight, I wish I had signed up for rehab much earlier.

CHAPTER 14
Lyme Disease

Attending Rehab was the best decision I ever made. By November of 2011, I was living free without pain medication. I was clean for Fiona's 1st birthday and our family seemed to be getting closer. '**Mommy was back**,' and life was getting better by the day. It felt so good to achieve what I had once believed to be unachievable. My perception of the world was starting to clear, and everything seemed so different. It saddens me that I did not get help earlier, and I will always regret the stress I caused my family. I am so grateful for their ongoing support and for being there when I came out on the other side.

People often ask me how I managed to get off the Norco without experiencing the dreaded withdrawal effects. When you are trapped by the reigns of addiction, it is hard to imagine a life without meds. The doctors at Rehab tapered me down at such a slow pace that I barely noticed the change. My body was adjusting and readjusting every step of the way, and although slow, the method worked. I had gotten used to taking eight Norco tablets per day before I went to Rehab. At first, my dosage got reduced to seven and a half tablets per day for five consecutive days. It was then further reduced to seven per day for five days, then six and a half per day for five days, then six, then five, and so on. Eventually, I reached a point where I was no longer taking Norco, and the only thing left to do was to continue not taking it.

Despite this method proving successful for me, <u>do not assume this will be the same for everybody.</u> I do not recommend this method of how I got tapered down. Get advice from your doctor to find the best tapering method for you or connect with me for a friendly ear and guidance.

I learned so much about myself at Rehab and gained an immense amount of invaluable knowledge relating to lifestyle choices and natural healing. I was so happy to be functioning again and will be forever grateful for the transformation.

However, I do still have unanswered questions:

- As a nation, why are we not taught about natural and free healing methods early in school?
- Why is natural healing not the first option offered to us by the so-called experts during our time of desperation?
- As a nation, why are we falsely informed that prescribed pain medications are not addictive?

Many millions of people, of all ages, are addicted to pharmaceutical drugs, which are issued to them legally by medical professionals. There are so many adults and children living in a state of depression, feeling isolated, lonely, numb, and suicidal. The medical authorities involved in allowing this vicious cycle to continue within our communities, must be made to stop, but how? Despite feeling angry and disappointed in our 'healthcare system,' I was happy to be clean and even happier to be alive.

My mission is to raise awareness for those still suffering. People who suffer from chronic pain, illness, or mental instability often need support in learning how to manage their lives. In many cases, the help is available without needing high doses of strong medication.

We need a health system that promotes natural healing!

One morning, my youngest boy Kane, who was aged thirteen at the time, came downstairs to leave for school and said to me, ***"Mom, I have the worst headache I have ever had in my life."*** I took a deep breath, asked him a few basic questions, and rushed him to the Emergency Room where

I had hoped to receive some guidance. I had never seen my son in so much pain before and had never heard him say anything like that. All I could think about was a possible brain tumor or aneurysm! He was in agony. The doctor carried out a CT scan on his brain, and after that was done and reviewed, he came in to deliver the results. Naturally, I was expecting an explanation for Kane's sudden and very intense pain, but instead, he informed us that everything appeared normal, and that Kane was just suffering from a migraine. He prescribed a selection of pain medications to help Kane's immediate situation and instructed us to follow up with our pediatrician.

As time passed, his headaches continued to return, and after numerous visits to the Emergency Room and his pediatrician, Kane was officially diagnosed with Chronic Daily Migraines. His pediatrician referred us to a neurologist since none of the medications she prescribed for him worked. We set up an appointment with the neurologist right away. It pained me so much to see my son taking pain medication, but I could not deprive him of the instant relief it offered. We had no idea what was wrong with him. The neurologist examined Kane and prescribed various migraine medications, but nothing worked. Kane couldn't go to school because the pain was so bad it was blinding him. He stayed on his bed, in the dark, day after day, unable to play video games, unable to watch TV, and unable to hang out with friends. As his mother, I cannot tell you how this affected me. I was beginning to think that since the migraine medications were not working, maybe it was not a migraine. I tried all the basic natural solutions to reduce the effects of migraines, including eliminating sugar, dairy, and gluten from his diet. I even tried herbal supplements but still, nothing helped.

I was not going to stop researching and seeking out help for my son. I wanted to know the cause of his pain, and to achieve that, I needed the right medical specialist. I was accused of doctor-shopping and being an attention seeker by family members, but that was not going to stop me either. Although the false accusations caused us a lot of sadness and tore the family apart, nothing could stop me from finding the right help for my boy. In order to help him heal, we had to know what was wrong.

I was not going to stop until Kane was better.

I took him to an ophthalmologist to check his eyes. I then booked an appointment with a neurologist described as the 'best in the country'. After several more weeks of trying different migraine medications, he told me, *"I think your son is depressed and does not want to go to school."* That neurologist then sent us to see a child psychologist who stated that our son was not depressed but sick. She then referred us to a pediatric neurologist from the Children's Hospital, who also tried various migraine medications, scans, and x-rays. Following that, Kane was admitted to the hospital to have a spinal tap performed. The reason for a spinal tap is to check the pressure of the spinal fluid on the brain (cerebral pressure). They do this by removing the fluid through a hollow needle inserted into the lower spine. He said the results were 'high' and concluded that this was the cause of Kane's headaches.

The diagnosis: Pseudotumor Cerebri

Pseudotumor Cerebri is when the brain thinks it has a tumor when it does not. It is a brain condition that causes the same symptoms as a tumor and produces excess spinal fluid as a direct result. Although devastated and shocked, we were thankful to have received an answer. The doctor recommended putting a shunt in his brain, with a tube attached to it, to drain the excess cerebral spinal fluid into his stomach. This guy was talking about major surgery!

As there are so many factors to consider before a spinal tap can be performed, my husband and I decided that we needed a second opinion. We wanted to make sure the diagnosis we had received was the correct diagnosis. Do not let anyone tell you this is *"doctor shopping."* This doctor wanted to perform life-altering brain surgery on my little boy. I could not allow my son to go through brain surgery under the instruction of just one doctor's opinion, not after my experience. My instinct was strong, and I knew something was not right about the guidance we were receiving.

It turns out, the diagnosis was <u>wrong</u>.

We took Kane to a different neurologist who specialized in Pediatric Pseudotumor Cerebri, and he confirmed that his cerebral pressure was normal and that he did not require major surgery. I was so relieved, but back at square one again. His 'chronic migraines' continued, and we still had no idea why this was happening.   During that time, my older son Kyle was dating a girl with Lyme disease, and while talking to her mom one day, she asked me if Kane had been tested for Lyme disease. It was probably the only test we had not tried. I carried out some research and booked an appointment with a Lyme disease specialist. He sat with us for over an hour asking Kane about his symptoms and me about his history. He was already sure that Kane had Lyme disease before even doing the tests. He proceeded to order a series of tests, and we waited patiently for the results.

One week later, we received a call from the doctor, and not only did the blood tests come back positive for Lyme disease, but it turns out that Kane had also developed several coinfections as a direct result of it being left untreated for so long. His numbers were off the charts.

We finally had the answer.

The doctor prescribed Kane several rounds of antibiotics and antiviral medications, and within a few weeks, Kane's headaches were gone! Currently, there is no cure for Lyme disease. Parasites hide and reproduce in the muscle tissue throughout the body, attacking different parts of it. Kane will still suffer debilitating headaches, although nothing like before. He chooses no pharmaceuticals for pain, instead choosing to lie down in the dark until it passes. He has some bad and some good days, but overall, he is much better than he was.

Always trust your parental instinct and do not give up on getting the answers your child deserves.

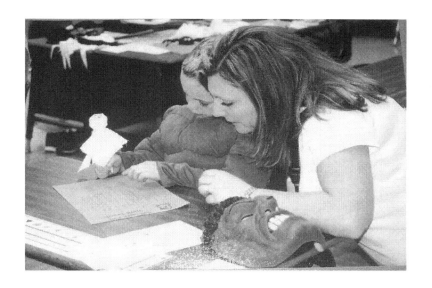

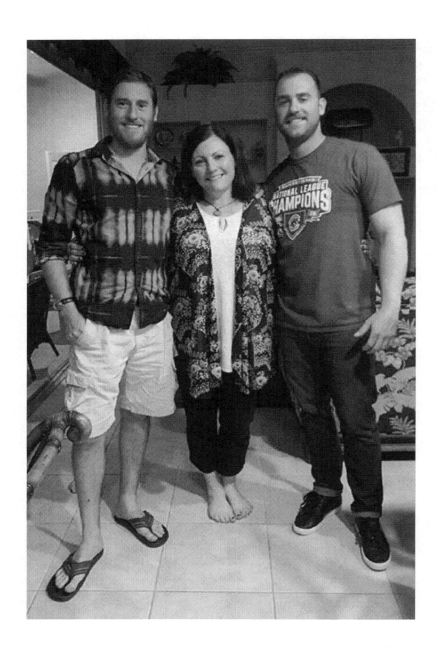

CHAPTER 15

Holistic Health

With every high comes a low. Although my life had changed and I was doing well after completing Rehab, my son was still suffering from Lyme disease, and his headaches, although less, were still causing him pain. I felt helpless as his mother and had no idea about what I could do to make his life better. It was not long before his social circle began to disintegrate. He became unable to attend school, go out with his friends, go to the movies, or invite them to visit our home. It was not an easy time for him. The strangest thing was, I knew how it felt to lose friends because of not being able to leave the house. We provided the best support we could for him, and although it was hard, he fought and fought. His headaches have lessened significantly since receiving the proper medical treatment, but he still gets them when he is exposed to high temperatures for long periods, and when he physically overexerts himself. Caring for my son led me to want to learn even more about **how food affects our bodies**. I had successfully put my Rheumatoid Arthritis symptoms into remission by following a healthy lifestyle and practicing what I had learned during my time in Rehab. I applied the same knowledge, where suitable, to Kane's well-being, and tried to keep us all on a healthy path as much as I could. I had a strong urge to share my newly found knowledge with the world and decided to begin training to become a certified Holistic Health Coach.

After plenty of research, I found an online school in New York that offered this certification. I knew that it required my complete dedication, but I was ready for the challenge. I registered with the course in late 2011 - with a sheer determination to succeed. I worked hard, but towards the end of my course, the dreaded back pain returned.

It could not have come at a worse time.

I was in the middle of studying for my exams, and the last thing I needed was more pain! It was ruthless, unbearable, and traveled down my side and through my legs. I began to feel scared about why this was happening and feared how it would affect my exam results.   Another CT scan led to another diagnosis. This time, the level under my two-level spinal fusion had herniated, causing the spinal cord to pinch as a result. The questions running through my mind were overwhelming. What was I supposed to do? Do I accept pain medication as a short-term solution and complete my course? Do I refuse the meds, quit the course, and head straight for surgery? What about my future as a Health Coach?

Stuck between a rock and a hard place, I decided to quit the course and head straight for surgery.

When I told my school mentor of my decision to quit, she would not have any of it. She discussed the pain medications at length with me and advised me to complete the course. She shed new light on my situation and reminded me that I was not the same person as before. Accepting pain meds to relieve immediate pain is very different from walking blind into an addiction. They should be taken solely for the purpose intended and viewed as a temporary solution. I knew what they could do to a person, but I was stronger this time, equipped with tools, too afraid of becoming a zombie, and too alert to allow myself to get addicted. I had very mixed feelings about taking them, but something felt different. They say knowledge is power and I think I agree. She gave me the confidence I needed to finish my course. I accepted her advice, thought mind over matter, and studied hard to achieve my goal. To this day, I am grateful for the faith she had in me and will always appreciate her honesty.

I passed with flying colors, with Honors, and became a Certified Holistic Health Coach in 2012.

After my graduation, I set up my own Holistic Health Coaching business. I created a new website detailing my services and began marketing the website online. My focus was to help people suffering from chronic pain and illness. It turned into a successful Chronic Pain & Illness support group that I managed out of a local coffee shop. I worked with a few clients and successfully helped them to achieve a healthier and more productive lifestyle.

Our financial situation was improving steadily, and we lasted in the rental property for two years. Then, Rob learned of a new government program designed to help people who had suffered a catastrophic loss and required assistance for a mortgage. We took the necessary steps to find out more about the program and, unbelievably, found ourselves in a position, once more, where we could buy a house! Naturally, I had concerns about building up more debt, but my husband insisted that we *"go for it."*
This is why I have such a deep love for Rob. He makes us believe, encourages us to push the boundaries, and is not afraid of embracing change. He is the reason we take steps outside of our comfort zone. In April 2013, I underwent surgery once more. It was difficult to accept this was happening again, but I fought hard not to let it get me down. It was a one-level spinal fusion surgery, but this time it was performed through my back.

The surgery was a success.

I still needed a blood transfusion, but after that, everything seemed trun smoothly. Due to the lifestyle changes I had adopted, I felt stronger and more able to deal with the effects of the surgery. The hard work that I had invested in myself was finally paying off. A consistent nutritional diet, healthy living, regular exercise, and a positive mindset had set me up for this journey of self-healing.

My immune system was doing its job.

The recovery period was flawless and easy, and I immediately stopped taking all pain medication. It was then when I truly realized how important it is to be fit and able, all the time. If I had learned the benefits of leading a natural and healthy lifestyle from a young age, I could have achieved a much healthier life in the long run.   By November 2013, Kyle had moved to Minnesota, Kane was homeschooling, and we had moved into our new home, in a completely new area. It was a fresh start for all of us.

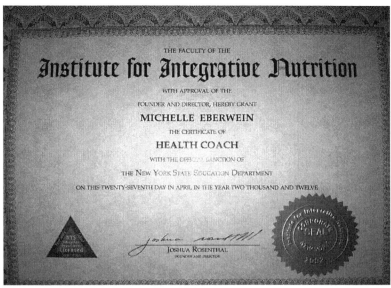

THE FACULTY OF THE

Institute for Integrative Nutrition

WITH APPROVAL OF THE

FOUNDER AND DIRECTOR, HEREBY GRANT

MICHELLE EBERWEIN

THE CERTIFICATE OF

HEALTH COACH

WITH THE OFFICIAL SANCTION OF

THE NEW YORK STATE EDUCATION DEPARTMENT

ON THIS TWENTY-SEVENTH DAY IN APRIL IN THE YEAR TWO THOUSAND AND TWELVE

JOSHUA ROSENTHAL
FOUNDER AND DIRECTOR

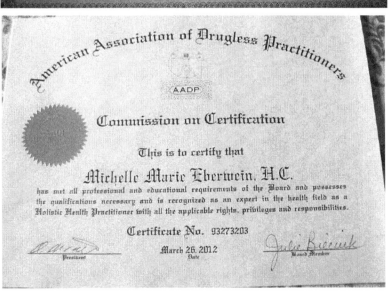

American Association of Drugless Practitioners

AADP

Commission on Certification

This is to certify that

Michelle Marie Eberwein, H.C.

has met all professional and educational requirements of the Board and possesses the qualifications necessary and is recognized as an expert in the health field as a Holistic Health Practitioner with all the applicable rights, privileges and responsibilities.

Certificate No. 93273203

March 26, 2012
Date

President

Board Member

CHAPTER 16
Natural Healing

Christmas of 2013 was approaching fast, and we were all looking forward to spending it in our new home. Despite the ongoing dilemmas and challenges, we were happy. I had adopted many lifestyle changes to help me deal with the pain, using natural methods, and it finally felt as if I was winning. Unfortunately, whenever I experienced feelings of success, I always found myself thinking that they were too good to be true. Waiting for the pain to return, I was pleasantly surprised when life continued to improve. I was so glad not to be on the meds anymore.

My main goal, every day, was (and still is) to keep the pain away. I made significant changes to my routine and diet. Every morning, I start my day with an ice-cold glass of water to wake my body up and get my organs moving. I include fresh citrus fruits in the water, especially lemon, which contains high levels of Vitamin C and natural antioxidants. These provide anti-inflammatory benefits, which help to reduce internal and external swelling. Drinking lemon juice in the morning aided me to put my Rheumatoid Arthritis into remission. Combatting the swelling, first thing in the morning, after a good night's sleep, helps to prepare my body for the day ahead. If there is one positive lesson that I have gained from living with chronic pain, it is to eat properly. You are what you eat and can reduce the pain by eating the right foods. Sugar, vegetable oils, processed meats, and other inflammatory foods are almost certain to increase the pain. Learning about nutrition has gifted me a whole new perspective on life. If you want to build and maintain a strong immune system, diet is everything. Adding natural supplements to your diet such as turmeric, ginger, fish oil, and multivitamins, also helps to reduce inflammation. Nowadays, at home, our diet is based around non-chemical foods, fruits, and vegetables.

Another powerful healer that we must not forget about is the sun. It seems hard to believe that spending time in the sun strengthens your immune system, but it does. It provides a natural source of Vitamin D, which plays a significant role in regulating calcium and phosphorus levels in the blood. Both calcium and phosphorus are crucial for maintaining healthy bones and, for me, are two of the most effective natural healers.

I tried various natural pain relief creams as well, but the most helpful cream I found was Topricin Pain Cream. It is a coconut-based moisturizing cream blended with natural homeopathic medicines and is made entirely from plants. It helps to relieve pain and heal the damage that causes discomfort in the joints, nerves, and muscles. I will always recommend this healing cream as it is 100% non-chemical. I still use it to target specific pain areas when I feel the pain increasing. Heating pads, ice packs, braces, and Epsom salts diluted in the bath, also reduce the pain being caused by Fibromyalgia. Essential oils are also a valuable addition to the mix. I use oils such as peppermint, citrus oils, and specialty blends created specifically to target pain and mental stability. These can be blended with a carrier oil and applied directly to the skin.

Now, while all the above certainly decrease pain levels and strengthen your immune system, without physical exercise incorporated into your everyday routine, you will struggle to keep the muscular pain away. The key for me to dealing with chronic muscular pain is to keep moving. Every morning, I allocate time to stretch and meditate. Not only does it cause my muscles to relax and become flexible after stiffening up during hours of sleep, but helps me to focus, clear my mind, and achieve a calm and well-balanced approach to my day. Of course, there are days when my body refuses to want to stretch, but if I can, physically, I will! Stretching every morning improves my range of motion and allows me more freedom of movement throughout the day. My posture has dramatically improved as a result, and so have my stress levels. It is always good to understand why you are doing something and how it helps you, physically and mentally.

Regular stretching improves blood circulation, which, in turn, increases blood flow to your muscles. This is vital for reducing soreness. During the exercises, I focus intently on the connection between Mind and Body and find huge benefits in taking the time to meditate before I embark on the next phase of my daily routine. Stretching, combined with good nutrition and a healthy lifestyle, has changed my life significantly. If I stop exercising for too long, my muscles seize up and feel like concrete.

Swimming is another excellent solution for building muscular strength and maintaining flexibility. The feeling of weightlessness affords me immediate temporary relief, and I can stretch my body in ways that are otherwise impossible out of the water. Massages too; if you can find a good massage therapist, I highly recommend a professional massage every couple of weeks. Regular massages help to keep the muscles loose around your spine, which is incredibly effective for reducing soreness and feelings of tenseness.

It is hard to explain to someone suffering from chronic pain that these natural healing methods work as a long-term solution. If they are on a course of strong pain medication, you may have a difficult time getting through to them, and it may seem like they have no interest in what you have to say. It took for me to attend Rehab and specialist courses to find out the benefits of good nutrition and exercise. Do not give up on them. They are most likely listening to every word you say.

Your words of encouragement could well be the reason they finally decide to stop.

During my addiction, I did not have the energy to converse with anybody. I did not want to hear about what I should be doing or what I was doing wrong. At the same time, being alone with my thoughts was also something I wanted to avoid. Owning a pet helped me in so many ways. Boo was always there when I felt alone, so, I was never really alone. She kept me going with her unconditional love and affection, especially when I could not open up to my loved ones. I did not need to explain myself to her. She was there when I felt suicidal, late at night, when I woke up in the morning and needed a reason to smile, when I was alone at home, and when I cried in pain. I know that Boo played a big part in saving my life.

Everything I have learned about how to manage pain; I learned the hard way. If I had known then what I know now, my way of dealing with everything would have been very different.

It was not until I began to understand the pharmaceutical industry and the seriousness of the corruption inside our medical healthcare system that I woke up to realize what was happening to me. It is so important to me to share my experience with the world. If I can help one person who feels lost and without direction, then it is worth doing. I want you to know that there are ways you can survive this without making any dramatic or bad decisions.

I will listen to and help you if you feel alone with nobody to turn to.

Likewise, if you know someone experiencing chronic pain, depression, or medication addiction, let us help them out of it. Feeling like a useless burden on your support circle is one of the most dangerous emotional states you can find yourself experiencing. Once you begin to feel like a burden, it is so easy to feel unwanted, and this can lead to more isolation, a stronger addiction to escapism through pain medication, and, eventually, suicide. During my addiction, I believed that my family would be better off without me and that they no longer needed me at home. I felt like this, not because of my family's actions, but because of my psychological wellbeing (or lack of it)!

I needed to feel useful, somehow.

Hope in Bracelets was born in 2014 and remains one of my best creations. I began to make awareness bracelets for unknown illnesses and incurable medical conditions. Following this, I launched an Etsy store and still sell them there today with a percentage of my earnings going to charity. The reviews I receive give me so much purpose. The ethos behind this project was always to raise awareness, one bracelet at a time, but then I started to feel that I was making a difference in people's lives. My physical ability was restricted but using my hands to create something meaningful was so rewarding. There are always ways for us to occupy our minds and do good. Every one of us has the power within us to change, and if we can learn to channel our inner fears and frustrations correctly, life can change for the better, in the blink of an eye. I could barely walk or dress myself when Hope in Bracelets took off, but I could use my hands, and that is what I did.

Lastly, I just want to remind you briefly about Biofeedback, a mind body technique that involves using auditory or visual focus to gain control over your pain. I mentioned earlier in the book that I was skeptical about attending this class at rehab, but it turned out to be one of the most important lessons I received. By distracting your brain from the pain, you can reduce heart rate, blood pressure, and muscle tension. A series of mental exercises involving visualization taught me how to rise above my physical location into another place. It took me a while to accept this could work in the long run.

An example would be when they told me to visualise the following, *"...in a field of flowers, the wind is blowing lightly, the sun is shining. Feel the warm sun on your face as you inhale the scent of the flowers,"* and it continued.

By playing this entire story and visualizing it in your mind, your brain gets distracted, and you forget about the pain. I know it is hard to believe; I thought it was corny and had a small attitude with the Biofeedback Therapist, but I gave it a chance, and it worked. I was grateful to have another management tool that did not involve pharmaceutical drugs. I was learning to manage the pain using nonchemical solutions, and it was working.

CHAPTER 17
Freedom

Six weeks later, the pain returned with a vengeance. I can only describe it as large shards of broken glass being stabbed repeatedly into my right leg and foot. It was agonizing! I booked an appointment with my doctor and immediately had another x-ray and CT scan. The results showed that scar tissue had grown back under the nerve roots in my lower spine! I was told this was a common negative side effect of spinal fusion surgery. So, why wasn't I informed of this possible side effect before the surgery took place? More visits to the doctor later revealed that the scar tissue was growing back thicker, and, within two months, had formed around my spine, as well as my nerve roots. You could not make it up. I was told that surgery was required to remove the scar tissue, but I could not possibly undergo surgery every time it grew back. The thought of having surgery every few months to manually remove it was not a solution to my problem. The surgeon prescribed steroids to reduce the inflammation and offered me a separate course of strong pain meds to help me cope. Feelings of resentment, fear, and anger, had me teetering on the edge of a very dark space. Why was I being subjected to more pain? Why, when life was improving so much for all of us, did this have to happen? It was exhausting, but things were different this time. It felt good to be in a state of awareness and trusted myself to be guided by my instinct.

I firmly declined the pain medication.

Addiction was not a risk I was willing to take. Rob had recently changed profession, and we were required to wait three months before the health insurance coverage became effective. I could not schedule the recommended surgery straight away, so I dedicated myself to another journey of self-healing through healthy living. My diet was clean, controlled, and tailored to keep my immune system strong. I used every pain management tool I knew and followed a strict routine to keep my brain occupied until the day for surgery arrived.

I had done it again. Through a tailored diet and exercise routine, I had stayed off the meds until the big day arrived.

Upon arriving at the medical center, they informed me that the surgery would be a straightforward process called a bi-lateral foraminectomy. The surgeon planned to cut open a previous incision in my back to four inches, so that he could remove the scar tissue away from the nerve endings. He told me that it would prevent any additional scars from forming. Truthfully, I did not care about my scars; they were and still are all that remains of my battle wounds; my roadmap of life per se. Once again, I put all my trust in the medical 'experts' and trusted them to operate on me.

The next thing I remember was waking up and feeling the most excruciating pain. I tried, several times, desperately, to try and get some instant pain relief, but due to low blood pressure, they declined. The doctor came over to inform me that my body had reacted badly to the surgery and that *"things had just not gone to plan."* He had no idea why my body was reacting the way it was and decided that I needed a blood transfusion to aid in a successful recovery. Staying in the hospital for five more nights was worth it if it meant stopping the pain!

Despite everything, the nurses were kind, and thankfully, the blood transfusion was a success. I was finally able to return home. The pain had reduced to a more tolerable level, allowing me to sit, stand, walk, and move around freely. I accepted a very low dosage of pain relief medication to help me recover from the surgery, and all I had to do was focus on achieving a fast and flawless recovery. It felt good to be back at home with my family, Boo, and all my creature comforts.

As the weeks and months passed, I could feel myself improving a little more each day. This progress continued until six months later when a crippling pain took over my entire body.

The scar tissue had grown back, again.

I could not take any more of this torture, and I needed help, fast. My doctor offered me a low dosage of Norco as a temporary solution to relieve some of the pain. It is exactly what I needed, but I had been addicted to Norco before. I knew the dangers this drug presented. After thinking hard about what to do; I accepted a 5mg dosage to help me get by while I explored my options. The pain was still so unbearable that I ended up taking various other pain relief injections and nerve medications as well. Although disappointed in myself, I felt that I was making controlled, informed decisions.

The next pain management doctor I got referred to wanted to take me off all pain medication for a full twelve months. He said this would help to identify the baseline of my pain and recommended implanting a Spinal Cord Stimulator. As he talked me through the process, it sounded like something I would consider, but I was not ready for another surgery just yet. The thought of anyone implanting anything on my spinal cord was hard to fathom. He was quite forceful about me having it, which made me uncomfortable in his presence. To my surprise, when I declined the surgery, he said he no longer wanted to care for me. I decided he was not the right doctor and continued my quest to search for alternative treatments.

Eventually, I found a new pain doctor who had some new ideas about pain relief. She was easy to talk to and showed a great understanding of my circumstances. She agreed that implanting a Spinal Cord Stimulator was the best long-term solution, but took things very slowly, and at a pace, I felt comfortable with. Her first plan was to perform a procedure called Lysis of Adhesions. It is where a saline solution is injected into the scar tissue using a needle. Studies have shown that the scar tissue breaks up and gets absorbed by the body, freeing up the encased nerves and putting an end to the pain. To me, it sounded like the perfect solution, but, unfortunately, my insurance company deemed it an experimental procedure and refused to authorize payment for it.

Instead, they suggested I take Morphine.

My doctor decided against Morphine and offered me a different type of pain medication designed to intercept the pain signals to the brain, resulting in decreased pain and no brain fogginess. I remember a similar type of medication that was released a while back called Opana, but people started crushing it, injecting it, and inhaling it for recreational purposes. It was pulled off the market in the end. I got prescribed Nucynta ER (extended-release tablets), which are contained in a drug-resistant shell to ensure they cannot be tampered with, and they helped me a lot, for a while, anyway.   By April of 2015, I was bed-bound on most days. I was taking pain medication, but nothing was changing. Rob and I discussed my options repeatedly and attended numerous meetings with the pain doctor. Rob was in favor of the Spinal Cord Stimulator, but the thought of the surgery made me feel sick. I could not face another major surgery. Even the simplest of surgeries had caused so many setbacks, so the thought of another major surgery performed on my spinal cord was soul-destroying. My doctor spent a lot of time explaining the procedure to me and agreed that the Spinal Cord Stimulator was the best, most reliable long-term solution. After all that I had been through, did I want to do this? The only other option was to have a pain pump installed.

I was tired of feeling useless and Kane was struggling to keep up with his homeschooling. Unless I was next to him, pushing him to complete the work, he took so long, and the work did not get done; he was reliant on me sitting with him. I carry tremendous guilt where his education is concerned. I feel that I could have done more to help him. I did not have the energy to provide the moral support he deserved, and the pain was so severe that I could not focus on helping him complete his schoolwork. I wish I had been stronger and healthier to help him achieve his goals, but I struggled to even get myself out of bed. He decided to quit homeschooling. There was not much we could do other than, respect his decision.

In the end, Rob persuaded me to proceed with the Spinal Cord Stimulator.

I scheduled a consultation to find out everything there was to know about this device. We put all our questions to the doctor, and she cleared up any uncertainties. It all begins with a trial, whereby they insert a temporary stimulator for seven days to see if you are a suited candidate. I felt petrified by the thought of having a long cord threaded up from my tailbone to the middle of my spine and placed on top of my spinal cord! It certainly was not an easy decision to make, but it got easier as I thought of my family. My boys needed their mom, as my husband needed his wife.

I had to put my fear aside and get on with it.

We booked a date for the trial placement to take place. On the morning of the surgery, I was nervous. I kept thinking 'this has to work,' and as we arrived at my doctor's office, I remember feeling ready to start a brand-new chapter. Please, God, let this work!   I felt an almighty sense of relief as the sedatives flowed through my veins - it was too late to turn back now. After forty-five minutes, the device had been inserted, and without incident. I counted that as a small win. Once I had woken up and regained full consciousness, the moment finally arrived for us to test the device. The doctor, with a smile on her face, turned the Spinal Cord Stimulator to ON.

First, I moved my legs; I stood up, walked around, sat down, and still, no pain. I laughed, I cried, and, carefully, continued to move around. Still, no pain.

For the first time in two years, I felt no pain whatsoever.

An overwhelming wave of relief, gratefulness, and freedom consumed me. It felt so alien being able to move around without any restrictions. I could not believe the result.

The pain was gone.

Of course, I often think about why I had not agreed to the stimulator before. Sometimes, we make decisions out of fear that can hold us back from getting better, but you need to be physically and mentally ready to take on any major surgery. I needed to get there first.

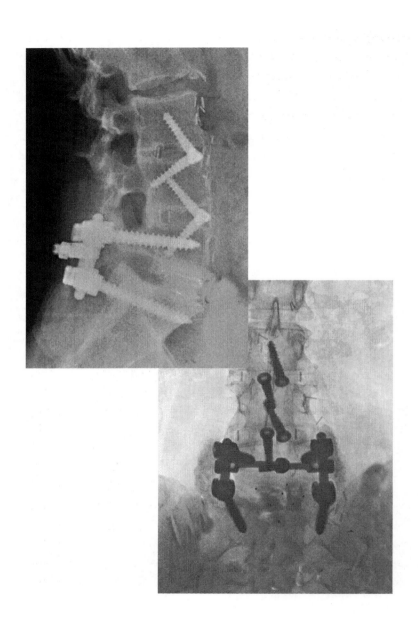

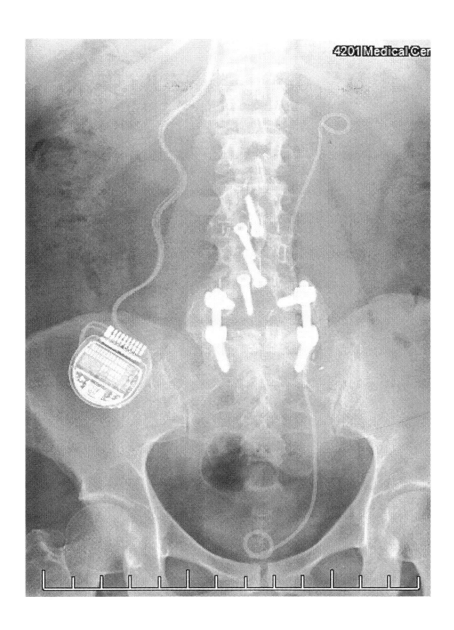

CHAPTER 18
Statute of Limitations

Had I been blessed by a guardian angel? It certainly felt like it! Every morning, I would wake up, shower, and dress. Making breakfast and carrying out household chores had become enjoyable tasks, and I felt grateful to be able to do them. I could move around and spend time with my boys without feeling pain. I could cook homemade meals, enjoy my evenings with Rob, and be the wife and mother I intended to be. I could visit my sister, go to the shops, and function like a healthy human being. Adjusting to this new way of life, however rewarding, did not come without its challenges. I had difficulty accepting that the pain would never return. After years of thinking about when the next trauma would arise, it was hard to get out of that mindset.

I focused on getting back to work as soon as possible. I could not wait to be back in employment. As I started looking into all my options, I came across Rita Hickman, a Shiatsu Massage Expert and Life Coach. It was during the summer of 2015, and Rita was looking for help with secretarial and marketing tasks at her venue, which just so happened to be the perfect venue for the type of health and wellness classes I wanted to hold. As I arrived to meet Rita for the first time, she greeted me with open arms into one of the most Zen spaces imaginable. I will always remember the smell of Lavender in the air and how I immediately felt comforted. We got to know each other, and it was not long before we had reached a mutual agreement. The deal stated that I would help Rita with marketing tasks in return for a small payment and access to her venue for holding my classes. We were both happy with the arrangement, and I started soon after. I knew instinctively that this was a good connection, but I had no idea that it would lead to creating some of the best memories in my new health coaching career.

Rita's space is in downtown McHenry, Illinois. Going to work there made me feel active and useful; it felt so good to leave home and go to work! Admittedly, I was apprehensive about starting my new classes, as I had never hosted a class before, and my nerves were getting the better of me. Thankfully, Rita stayed with me and showed me how it was done. I went from being incredibly shy to a confident speaker in no time at all, and that is when I learned that it is perfectly OK to be who you are. When you finally stop caring about how others perceive you and focus on being your best self, you realize the true meaning of the word 'Freedom.' It took a few good sessions before I finally let go and allowed myself to shine. Rita gave me the confidence to communicate concisely and effectively and to use these skills in sharing my knowledge with others. She has a unique gift for helping people heal from past traumas and embrace the best version of themselves. I will always be thankful to Rita for helping me overcome my fears. I was progressing brilliantly and had experienced a significant transformation since working there.

There was, however, one thing concerning me.

It was a crippling left-sided flank pain that kept returning every few months. Every time I got booked in for a CT scan, the diagnosis was different. First, they said I had a kidney stone; then, a urinary tract infection; then, an ovarian cyst. The pain was so sudden that it had me doubled over and sometimes even vomiting. Then, after another CT scan, I received some clarity. As the ER Doctor entered my room in the hospital, I felt nervous. *"When did you undergo spinal surgery through your abdomen, Michelle?"* he asked excitedly. I told him it was in 2007. *"They left a surgical tool inside of you,"* he said. Straight away, I assumed it was a scalpel, a pair of scissors, or something sharp, but he described it differently. *"It looks like a sponge of some sort. I am waiting to speak to the head of the Radiology Department."*

They referred me to a surgeon for an emergency appointment, who confirmed that it was indeed a surgical sponge. He also said that since the sponge adhered to the iliac artery, *"there is no 'safe' way to remove it."* He believed that the surgery required to remove the sponge would be complicated and advised me not to have it removed. He also advised me to consult a vascular surgeon, which I did, immediately. The vascular surgeon concluded that if I tried to remove the surgical sponge from my body, I could surely die. He confirmed that I should *"never touch it!"*

How did this go unnoticed by the medical experts who had performed countless scans and x-rays on me? Had not one of them noticed something unusual? A surgical sponge, maybe? When we allow these people to anesthetize us and cut open our bodies, we do not expect them to leave surgical tools inside us. Since the surgery had taken place in 2007, I had had countless scans, and not one surgeon had mentioned the sponge. How was this possible? It was no pea-size object but a surgical sponge! The more I thought about it, the angrier I became. I started looking online to find others who may have experienced a similar situation and discovered so many cases of people feeling the same way as I did. Knowing you have an object in your body that is not meant to be there is unsettling, to say the least. How could I leave it in there? There must be a way to remove the sponge safely without risking my life.

I had to do something. The last thing I wanted to do was to start pursuing legal action, but they had just informed me that I would forever suffer pain as a direct result of another surgeon's mistake! If my only option was to pursue legal action, then that is what I was going to do. I consulted lawyers to find out my legal position. I refused to accept that they could make such a mistake and get away with it.

I had been told that I would eventually end up in a wheelchair with my condition. After reading about the settlements other people had received,

I thought we could put an end to our financial struggle. If I could win this case, I could finally invest in a better mattress, orthopedic shoes, and cover the travel costs I needed to see the most suited doctors for my medical conditions. I could also make our home wheelchair-accessible, ready for when that time came in my future.

But then we received a call from our attorney.

He told me he was unable to take my case because he simply would not win. Due to the surgery taking place in 2007, too much time had passed. It turns out, in Illinois, if a doctor leaves a tool inside you, you only have four years to take legal action. After the four-year period has passed, the surgeon then becomes protected and cannot be sued. It is called the Statute of Limitations.

Doctors pay a <u>lot</u> of money for this law to be in place.

I had no case, but I could not just give up and accept that I had to live with a surgical sponge causing me health issues for the rest of my life. I knew that, in some states, they have *'exemptions in their statute of limitations, which allow patients with unintentionally retained objects to file claims after the deadline.'* If we could achieve a change in the Illinois Law, this would result in a positive life change for thousands of people like me.

I contacted our State Representative and Senator. The response stated that unless I had a ton of money, I could never change the law. I collected over 3,000 signatures from Illinois residents, agreeing that our Statute of Limitations Law needed to be changed, but none of this had the impact I was hoping it would have. I was, however, grateful when I received the call from ABC7 News Chicago, agreeing to cover my story. They launched an investigation and stated that *'medical mistakes are now estimated to be the third leading cause of death in the United States.'* They confirmed that my medical reports, since the surgery, *'... reveal that the experts knew something was inside her that shouldn't have been. In radiology lingo, an 'irregular high-density material.'*

The documentary also revealed that I am not the only one living in the dark. *'In Illinois, these sometimes deadly, serious mistakes are supposed to be reported to the state, but the I-Team has learned that hasn't been happening. According to the Illinois Department of Public Health, 'the legislative budget impasse has stalled our ability to sign a contract and pay a vendor to create an electronic reporting system.' At this time, hospitals are not reporting these events. The joint commission which accredits hospitals does keep track of items left inside surgical patients, telling the I-Team it happens roughly 2,000 to 4,000 times each year in the United States. But reporting to the commission and other agencies is voluntary, so the numbers are estimates.'* The more I fought to get this story exposed, the more I realized the seriousness of this problem happening within the US justice system.

The documentary then introduced Dr. Ronald Wyatt, who was heading the safety investigations at the time. He stated that *'There is, we believe, significant under-reporting of all safety events,'* and that the *'... commission is working to change the culture.'* Wyatt went on to reveal that *'We have had care teams when we go through a root cause analysis say to us, 'I knew something was left behind, but I couldn't say so.'*

Imagine working in the medical sector and feeling silenced about something so important. In this case, something that was ruining my life and possibly my future. Unfortunately, despite the many scans, I did not learn about the object in time.

According to medical malpractice attorney, Bill Cirignani, also featured in the ABC7 Chicago news documentary, *'In Illinois, doctors and hospitals lobbied for a deadline, a drop-dead deadline after which they cannot be sued even if their patients never are aware, or never become aware of the injury after that, ... It doesn't matter that people saw it and didn't tell her, doesn't matter that she had pain and asked about it and no one uncovered it. In Illinois, after four years, she is out."*

To this day, I still have regrets for not asking for the detailed reports immediately after my ER visits. I never dreamt, in a million years, that our health service would go that far to deceive us. You would have thought I would have learned my lesson after my experiences.

Life continued, the pain came and went, and I focused on developing my career as a Health Coach. Rita and I had a great working relationship, which I found to be an excellent support.

I try not to dwell on the surgical sponge and do everything I can to distract myself from thinking about it. However, once again, I find myself living with the Sword of Damocles hanging over me. When will the pain return? How long will it be before another infection or disease develops because of this abnormal object resting on my organs? Being told you can never remove it is incredibly difficult to accept.

I take one day at a time, step by step, goal by goal. Writing this book has forced me to reflect on all the mistakes I have made and opened doors for me to share my experiences with others still trapped by the reigns of addiction and depression.

The lessons I have learned through personal experience are invaluable to me and anyone I can help along the way.

Below, you can clearly see the irregular high-density material, a.k.a surgical sponge!

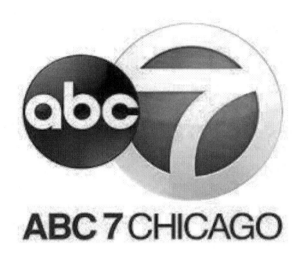

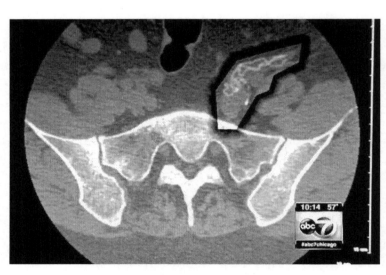

February 2, 2016

Ms. Michelle Eberwein
3407 W. Fairway Drive
McHenry, Illinois 60050

      RE: Eberwein
             Our File No. 15n-130

Dear Michelle:

Attorney Letter

We have now had an opportunity to complete our investigation of your potential claim against Drs. ███████ and ███████ in connection with the retained surgical sponge in your back. Unfortunately, we do not believe that under Illinois law we can bring a claim at this date as the statute of limitations has expired.

As we previously discussed, in Illinois a medical malpractice action must be brought within two (2) years of the date of malpractice or the date that you reasonably should have known of the malpractice. Under no circumstances can an action be brought more than four (4) years after the occurrence. The only potential exception is if there was fraudulent concealment on the part of the doctor who allegedly committed malpractice. As you know, it has been 8 ½ years since the initial surgery and 8 years since you last saw Dr. ███████.

Although the February 17, 2008, CT, references the possibility of a retained swab, there is no evidence to suggest that Dr. ███████ was aware of this finding or did anything to fraudulently hide this information from you.

Some states, Colorado and Connecticut for example, have exceptions in their statute of limitations which explicitly state that claims for injuries relating to retained objects fall outside the statute of limitations and statute of repose. Unfortunately Illinois courts have specifically stated that Illinois does not have such an exception, and that the statute of repose applies in retained object cases just like other cases. This result is undoubtedly frustrating, but based on our careful analysis, we do not believe that there is an applicable exception to the statute of limitations, notwithstanding the fact that she did not know about the retained object until last year. Thus, if we were to file a medical negligence complaint on your behalf, the Court would dismiss the case almost immediately.

55 West Wacker Drive • 9th Floor • Chicago, Illinois 60601 • Tel: 312-629-2900 • Fax: 312-629-2916 • Toll: 800-704-2900
www.mcnabolalaw.com

CHAPTER 19
Comfort Zone

The most valuable lessons I have learned are to trust your gut instinct and always be willing to make moves outside of your comfort zone. In the words of Albert Einstein, ***"Insanity is doing something over and over again and expecting different results."*** This resonates with me because being addicted to pain medication led me to repeat the same, negative pattern, day in and day out. You end up in a rut and echo the very actions you know may kill you in the end. It takes a lot to accept this truth before you do something about it; something inside you has got to want to change.

When I finally realized I needed professional help, I did not sign up for Rehab straight away. How could I go from being a pill-popping recluse to socializing with people I had never met before in an unfamiliar environment? It took a lot for me to find the courage to get out of that headspace, but when I did, I realized everything was going to be okay. As I settled into my first class, it became obvious that I was exactly where I needed to be.

Making that initial move will always seem daunting at first. For me, the easiest way of handling this fear is to stop dwelling on that which has not yet happened. All those weeks spent worrying about whether I would fit in or not, or whether I would be able to cope with the symptoms of withdrawal; it was all irrelevant in the end. To overcome your fear of signing up for rehab, think only about the next step. Do not worry about what you may or may not be able to achieve; go online, find a rehab center in your area, make sure it suits your needs, and register. Then, focus on preparing for the first day.

All you need to do is show up; the rest will follow.

Back in 2003, three years before my accident, I was determined to pursue a career in the medical field. I was confident in my ability to succeed but attending classes was not something I felt comfortable with. It took a lot of working myself up before I finally signed up for a course at the community college to become a Certified Nursing Assistant. The thought of joining a class, and socializing with people I had never met before, was petrifying. Taking small steps, I went online, found a course, and registered. I spent the following weeks feeling anxious about what I had committed myself to, but I resisted the urge to cancel. After countless sleepless nights, the first day of school had arrived. I put on a brave face and walked into class with my head held high.

My favorite part of the course involved on-site training with groups of elderly people in a local nursing home. I remember being a little nervous at first, but deep down, I knew it was my time to shine. I got to know the patients and loved listening to their life stories and philosophies. Most of them had an optimistic view of the world and showed great appreciation for the care they received. Sadly, there were also a few patients who chose not to accept our help and who preferred to remain alone. I tried my best to respect their wishes and privacy and did everything in my power to help them from a distance. Degenerative diseases such as Alzheimer's can cause great frustration in sufferers and their families. I would always try to put myself in their shoes, but it is impossible to fully understand what they are going through. If I could help them find a reason to smile, that was the ultimate gift for me.

You might be wondering why I am reminiscing at this stage; it is because these memories have helped in shaping who I am today. Going back to school gave me confidence and purpose.

I graduated as a Certified Nursing Assistant in the summer of 2004 and went on to work for my friend's home healthcare business. Tasked with visiting patients in their homes, and helping in areas where they struggled alone, I still believe that kindness, compassion, and patience, offer most of what they need to feel better. Working with the elderly has and will always inspire me.

Now, thirteen years later, I was itching for a new challenge.

Having just recovered from the Spinal Cord Stimulator surgery, I felt the need to use what felt like a new lease of life. Fostering puppies, however adorable, just wasn't filling that void for me. I spent quite a few weeks pondering what to do with my future. The idea of working as a medical assistant in a doctor's office had always appealed to me. Once I get these ideas in my head, it is hard not to go along with them. Going through the same emotions as I did with the Nursing Assistant Program in 2003, I was just as fearful this time round, in 2017. The main difference was that I was in a different place this time, mentally, and physically. Repeatedly reminding myself that fear is just a state of mind, I went online, found a suitable course, and registered with a full-time career school to become a Certified Medical Assistant. Yes, I was old enough to be everyone's mom in the class, but we all got along great, and it felt good to be working towards something new and exciting.

While things were going well, it was around that time when my oldest son, Kyle, and his girlfriend Kalli, announced they would be leaving Illinois to start their lives in Florida. As much as I would have liked to have begged them to stay, I knew how important it was to let them go. It was just so hard to accept they would be living so far away. Rob and I discussed moving to Florida as well. Apart from being closer to our son, there were many health and lifestyle benefits to be had. One of them was the difference in the weather; winters in Illinois are long and harsh, with extremely low temperatures and snowstorms. Anyone with any type of arthritis or muscular pain will know how cold weather affects our bones and joints. The winters were unpleasant for Rob too, as he worked long hours at a local car dealership, which, even in a blizzard, did not close. Rob would be expected to drive to work in dangerous conditions and spend most of the day in the car sales lot, cleaning snow off the cars. Moving to Florida would mean living in a much better climate.

The only thing holding me back from agreeing to go was the thought of leaving my sister and niece. Fiona had become the daughter we had never had, but we missed our son terribly, and Kane missed his brother.

Immersed in my course and determined to graduate, I was about halfway through when a severe pain paralyzed the entire left side of my body. I then noticed blood in my urine, I panicked. Thankfully, my son was there and able to drive me to the Emergency Room. After a series of tests were carried out, the diagnosis was kidney stones. Not one, not two, not three but four! They had found four kidney stones. Can you imagine what went through my head? I remember the doctor telling me, ***"Michelle, you will need to have laser surgery to break up the stones. Then, a wire stent will be inserted up through your bladder, and urethra, to your kidneys, to make more room for the broken pieces of stone to pass through with the urine."*** I was in so much pain that I found it difficult to absorb what he was saying. Before I knew it, the nurses had taken me into a room and prepared me for surgery. Upon waking up, I was delighted to hear it had all gone smoothly and was sent home to recover. The only thing left to deal with was the excruciating pain that I felt every time I urinated. If you can imagine what peeing fire and shards of glass, feels like, that is what I was going through. Fortunately, it only lasted a couple of days.

As soon as I was able to, my focus shifted straight back onto my studies. I had already missed one full week of school and was afraid of falling behind. I studied from my bedroom and memorized all the chapters off by heart.

In May of 2017, I graduated as a Certified Medical Assistant with straight As and passed the National Test.

I had done it! I had become a Certified Medical Assistant! After applying for various jobs online, I secured a role as a Pediatric Medical Assistant not too far away from where we lived. Working with babies and children gave me such a sense of fulfillment, and so many reasons to smile.

I often think that if I cannot contribute to my surroundings and the people in it, then what is my purpose for being here? It works both ways; if I had not received ongoing and unconditional love from my closest friends and family members during my darkest moments and times of desperation, where would I be now?

I may not have seemed to be listening to or acting on their advice, but I was listening to every word, and acted in the end.

Do not give up on the people you love.

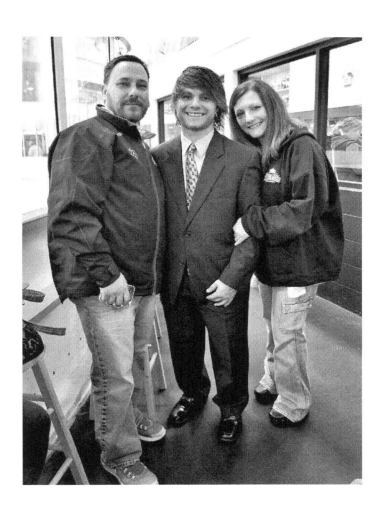

CHAPTER 20
Florida

By the end of the year, Rob and I had decided to sell our home and move to Florida. We had been talking about it for long enough and knew it was what we both wanted. We put together a plan allowing for six months for the house sale to complete, gave our employers ample notice, and secured a cute rental home in Cape Coral, Florida. You will not believe it when I tell you the house sold in one day! We were over the moon! By January of 2018, we were busy packing our belongings into the moving truck and getting ready to leave. Both the truck and our car were filled to the brim with bags and boxes. Our newly fostered pup, Jax, traveled in the truck with Rob, while Kane, Boo, and our cat, Fleury, came with me in the car. We had a thousand-mile journey in front of us, but we were ready. As we drove through the city, it all felt very surreal. I felt sad about leaving my sister and Fiona; it felt like it would be my last time there. On the plus side, I knew deep down that the positives outweighed the negatives and could not resist the excitement after we had left town.   I had spent the previous week preparing for the journey, to make it as enjoyable as possible for Rob and Kane. I had prepared a selection of their favorite snacks and drinks, and we stopped regularly to stretch our legs, switch the ice packs I was using on my back, and walk the dogs. They behaved wonderfully, and the entire journey from Illinois to Florida was flawless. As we arrived at our new home, Kyle, Kalli, my brothers, mom, and dad were all waiting to greet us.

We were so thankful to them for staying and helping us unload the truck. It immediately felt like home. That night, I remember lying in bed amongst the piles of boxes scattered throughout the room. All I could think about was how this was the ultimate fresh start for all of us. If I could leave all the medical drama behind in Illinois and start a new life with a strong and healthy approach, that is what I was going to do.

I immediately started looking for work.

Around a week later, I secured a position working as a Medical Assistant in a family practice nearby. Based in the doctor's office, I was thrilled to be working with such kind and caring people. Most of them were friendly and I honestly believed I would spend the rest of my career there. Nobody knew me or what I had been through, and no one needed to know. This was my chance to find myself again without people perceiving me as any less able than they. I was confident I could handle this role and excited to have gotten the job.   Unfortunately, being on my feet for 10-11 hours every day was eventually starting to take its toll on my health. Repeatedly bending over to help patients with their vitals and injections was turning into a painful experience. I ignored it and accepted a small dose of pain medication to help me function. By focusing all my energy on my new job, I had completely neglected the healthy lifestyle routine that had helped me manage the pain and put my Rheumatoid Arthritis into remission. My eating habits were nowhere near as controlled as they were before, and I was no longer dedicated to the morning stretching and meditation routines that had helped me to focus at the start of each day. I was finding it harder and harder to get up in the mornings and move around without crying. There were a couple of mornings where I cried all the way to work, the pain was so intense.

Admitting that I had done this to myself was not easy. I could not bear the thought of not working and had taken on too much too fast. I would return home from work each night, swallow a pain pill, and go straight to bed. I had neglected myself, and now I was paying the penalty. I submitted a request to my employer to see if it would be possible to decrease the number of hours I was working. They told me that I would lose my position working for the doctor I then worked with, which saddened me because we had a fun working relationship. But they offered me a part-time position working in the same office. I was delighted and immediately accepted. Sadly, as the weeks passed by, the pain was not going away or getting any easier to deal with. I went to see the neurosurgeon we referred our patients to, and, who after carrying out the relevant tests, said the pain was coming from lumbar level L2-L3.

"You will need another Spinal Fusion Surgery, Michelle," he said calmly.

How could I have allowed this to happen to myself? I considered every possible scenario relating to how I could have done things differently to avoid the repetitive strain on my spine. What if I had had the patients sit up on the exam table instead of bending over them, or turned down the extra hours working in different locations? What if I had been more committed to my health by waking up earlier to meditate and stretch? Would the pain have returned? Despite all the 'what ifs,' I had not done those things. With the help of pain medication, I continued working three days a week and dedicated the remaining four days to relaxation. I had hoped that that would be sufficient to help my body heal.

The routine continued for several weeks.

Every morning, I would take a pain pill and hope that by the time I was showered and dressed, I could physically sit and drive to work without suffering too much agony. I would get in the car with ice packs on my back and pray for the pain to go away. By the afternoon, it was most definitely time for another pain pill. After everything I had survived, it was not the life I wanted to be living. Taking pain meds was the last thing I wanted to be doing, but the thought of resigning was not an attractive option either. My job was everything to me.

Over time, the pain worsened, and I was becoming edgy. The medication was no longer numbing the pain and my handling of the patients was not what it used to be. Some of them would come in with simple, unoffensive complaints, and all I could think about was how foolish they were being. It was becoming impossible for me to keep up the façade of being this strong and pain-free woman. Due to constant feelings of anxiousness and fear, I started to withdraw from everyone.

In July of 2019, I was granted two weeks off work with a Doctor's Note. Unfortunately, by the end of the two weeks, I was still in no fit state to return to work, leaving me with no option other than to resign. It was such a tough decision to make but imagine how surprised I was when I called my boss to tell her, and she replied, ***"Honey, you've already been let go for not showing up to your shift."*** I was confused and asked her how she had reached that conclusion. It turns out, my supervisor, who had since been fired, had never told them I had been in daily contact with her or that I had found cover for my shift. Thankfully, I had all the texts and emails to prove it.

Always keep a written or digital record of any important communications you partake in, and do not lose your signed copies of documents. You never know when you might need them. In this case, it saved my reputation and possibilities of a future career there because I still hope to return to work there one day.

Since resigning from my role as Medical Assistant in August of 2019, I have not yet returned to work.

Not working in a fast-paced doctor's office has allowed me to live a healthier lifestyle and take much better care of myself. When the pain suddenly returns, I can react by lying flat on ice packs or the heating pad. I swim daily to keep my joints moving and muscles active. I do not believe I will ever be able to live entirely medication free, but I know my threshold and will never cross the line into another addiction.

I am brutally honest with my pain doctor; he understands that there will be no hard drugs or dosage increases unless all other options have been exhausted. I have not yet had the third Spinal Fusion Surgery and do not know if I ever will. Just the thought of going back into a surgery room is enough to start a panic attack.

Once the spine is manipulated, the surgeries will never end. There will always be another one as each disc degenerates.

More recently, over the last year and a half, we, like everyone, have been dealing with the devastating effects of the Covid-19 pandemic. When they first announced it, I was so worried for my family. My older son, Kyle, works in the medical field and was tasked with collecting and transporting Covid patients around. My husband works at a local car dealership, which is also considered an essential service during a pandemic. With Kyle and Kalli living two doors down from us in the same building, we are so used to seeing them regularly, but with both my husband and son going out to work each day, I was in a constant state of panic thinking about how they might get sick and bring the virus home.

Living in fear was not doing me any favors.

I turned off the TV and replaced it with my favorite music. Stretching, meditating, and swimming became a part of my daily routine. As my health improved, the pain became more manageable. Switching my focus onto healthy eating, I created a successful anti-inflammatory food program. In times like these, we need to keep strengthening our immune systems. I had all the time in the world to focus on healing and taking care of my family. I invested more time into designing my range of awareness bracelets and focused intently on finishing this book. It has not been easy, by any stretch of the imagination, but I am proud of myself for all that I have achieved and thankful to my support network for helping me achieve it. Not everyone is so lucky to have good people surrounding them, but if you are reading this, then I expect you know I am here for you.

Remember: I know how it feels to be isolated and alone; to be trapped by the reigns of addiction and depression; to feel like a burden on everyone around you. I continue to live with a surgical sponge inside my body, and I am told there is nothing I can do about it. It is impossible to know what my future holds at this stage, but I can confirm one thing; **a healthy life works wonders**.

Now, in 2021, I spend my days working from home on my awareness jewelry line and sharing the knowledge I have gained over the last fourteen years since the accident. I am also working on my second book, which goes into detail about the pain management tools I use, nutritional advice, and how to work towards a clear mind and body.

Some of my favorite memories ...

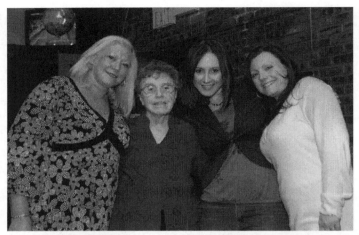

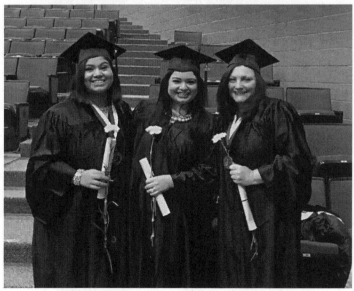

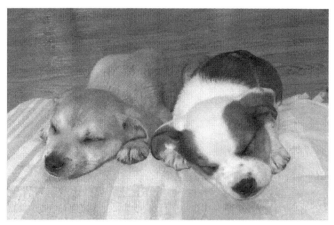

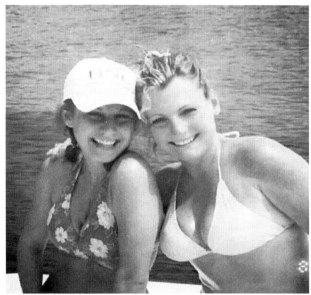

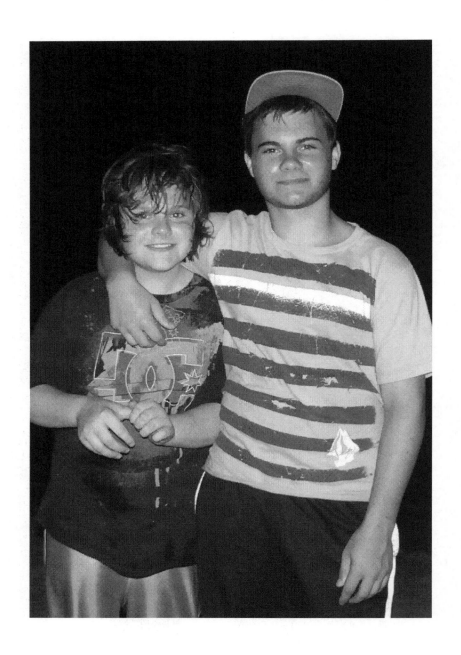

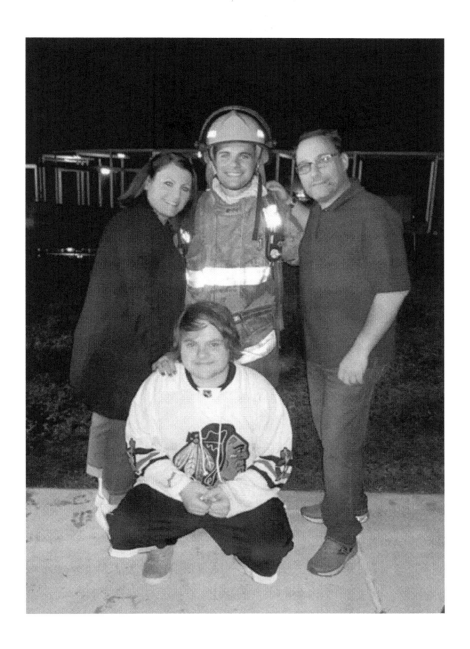

COMING SOON!

Turning Pain Into Strength II

Turning Pain into Strength II is the sequel to this book, and is where I will share with you, in detail, all the techniques I learned at Rehab and through my Nutrition and Health Coaching course. As someone who has lived with chronic pain for fifteen years and certified as a Medical Assistant, Holistic Health & Pain Coach, I will be revealing all the methods I use to ease the pain without the need for constant high dosages of pharmaceutical drugs, and a wealth of knowledge on the best lifestyle changes you can make to help keep the pain away.

The following subjects will be covered in detail:

- ✓ How to recognize the symptoms of Pain Medication Addiction
- ✓ How to deal with Addiction and how to end it
- ✓ Learn what Rehab offers and master the techniques
- ✓ Learn about Natural Healing methods and how to use them
- ✓ How to research Treatments and find the best one for you
- ✓ How to prepare for Surgery – mentally and physically
- ✓ How to embrace the Recovery Period and make it easier
- ✓ How to manage Rheumatoid Arthritis without Pain Medication
- ✓ How to manage Fibromyalgia without Pain Medication
- ✓ How to achieve a Healthier Lifestyle and Brighter Future

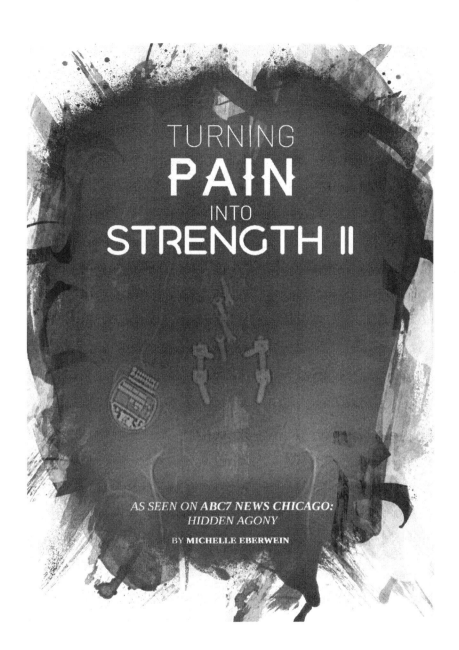

TURNING
PAIN
INTO
STRENGTH II

AS SEEN ON ABC7 NEWS CHICAGO:
HIDDEN AGONY

BY **MICHELLE EBERWEIN**

IN MEMORY OF
My Dad

My Dad dedicated his life to making sure that we, his family, never went without. He worked hard for many years in the Chicago Police Department and always made sure we had the best of everything, and more. He was a tough man who taught us that you never attempt anything unless you are ready to give it 100%. He always said, ***"With any major decision you make in life, weigh up the pros and cons, make your decision, and stick with it."*** Now that I am older, I understand how his tough approach to parenting made us strong and resilient adults.

At 72, my perfectly healthy Dad caught Covid.

On the 9th of March, he called me and left a voicemail. When I called him back, I remember my heart sinking to my stomach as he told me, ***"Shell, I got Covid."***

Barely three weeks had passed before he died. How did it happen so fast? In less than three weeks, my perfectly healthy Dad was taken from us forever. I now know how it feels to lose a parent; no matter what age you are, life becomes a little less certain. I listen to his last voicemail whenever I need to hear his voice.

It amazes me that people think this virus is fake or not serious. It destroyed my family and shredded our hearts into a million pieces.

It took me a while to realize that I was grieving a different dad than my siblings were. Looking back, he was still a kid himself when I came along, and his life was just getting started. My childhood memories are more of us spending time with my grandparents and uncles, going to many, many Chicago Cubs baseball games, attending big family dinners, taking trips up to our summer cottage in Wisconsin, and yearly trips to Florida.

My siblings, on the other hand, got a dad who was more involved in their lifestyles. He coached them in baseball, took them fishing, boating, and attended their afterschool activities and sporting events. The more I think about it, the more I find it fascinating how our family unit has developed over the years, and how my parents changed with the times.

As a grandfather, he loved his grandchildren and enjoyed attending Kyle and Kane's hockey games whenever he could. He was so proud of them and loved them dearly.

He may have had a hard time expressing his feelings to us, but he often talked about my siblings to me. Anytime my sister would post a photo of her girls online or send him a card with a photo on it, he would say, *"Isn't your sister such a great mom? Look how happy those girls always are."* He also often spoke to me about my brothers, John, and Anthony. He would say things like, *"John is such a hard-working, good man. He gets up before sunrise, every day, and goes to work. He works very hard, Michelle. And can you believe how he can cook? He is the best."* About my other brother, Anthony, he'd say, *"Anthony is such a great dad. To have a newborn while studying to become a Fire Fighter took a lot of patience and dedication, but it paid off. He really stepped up and grew up."* He said these things to me so many times and was so proud of all of us. He loved every single one of us dearly, and there is nothing he would not have done for his beloved wife, my mom.

Losing my Dad to Covid was the hardest thing I have ever experienced. He will never get to read my book, but I know he is watching over me, and I will continue to make him proud.

P.S. I will always remember the 5 Ps he taught us: Proper Planning Prevents Poor Performance. This applies to so many aspects of life.

THANK YOU FOR EVERYTHING DAD.

On the 28th of March 2021, I held his hand tightly as he took his last breath. I wanted him to read this book; he was not aware of everything I had been through. I wanted him to know that I never gave up and continue to fight every day.

IN MEMORY OF JOHN CARIOSCIA
NOVEMBER 16TH 1947 – MARCH 28TH 2021

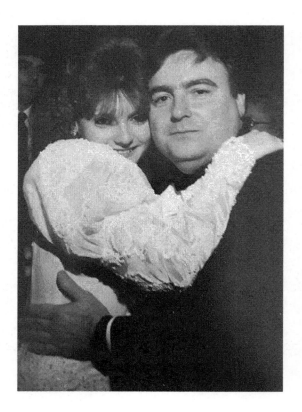

Hope in Bracelets

After being diagnosed with Rheumatoid Arthritis, Michelle learned there was very little information available about the disease. Most people believed it was the same as Arthritis and did not realize it is an incurable autoimmune disease. Michelle has pain & swelling in her joints, and is on weekly injectable, biologic medications to help control the disease. She started making bracelets to bring awareness to these medical conditions that have no cure and now accepts personalized orders from all over the world.

Testimonials:

"Thank you so much Michelle for another amazing piece. Everyone, including myself, is so blessed by one of your bracelets. I love giving them as gifts. God has blessed you with wonderful creative talents to help others even in the midst of your own suffering. You are very special. Thank you for making these beautiful inspiring bracelets. As a repeat highly satisfied customer, I know I will be back for more! Thank you & Blessings." **Patti**

"Love this beautiful bracelet!! Easy to get off and on especially with arthritic hands." **Kathy**

"I am in love with my bracelet. Not only is it a beautiful conversation piece, but it is made extraordinarily well. This is the only beautiful thing in my life that is related to CRPS. Thank you so much Michelle"
Danielle

"Michelle, thank you once again for making this special order for me and for also enclosing the beautiful personal card. That was so thoughtful, and I so appreciated it. Everyone that I've given one of your bracelets to has loved them! I'm sure my friend will love this special-order bracelet as well. Thank you for blessing so many of us with your talents, even as you suffer with your pain. You are truly appreciated!" **Anita**

...

To view a selection of my awareness bracelets, visit my Etsy store via my website at **TurningPainIntoStrength.com** or at **www.Etsy.com/shop/HopeinBracelets**

MAKING A DIFFERENCE
Together

"In order to raise awareness, it is really important for me to keep getting the word out. If you are a Bookseller, Podcast Host, Blogger or News Media outlet interested in being a part of this journey, please contact me. I look forward to hearing from you."

M. Eberwein

To contact Michelle Eberwein about covering her story, please send an email to **turningpainintostrength@gmail.com** or send a message via her website at **TurningPainIntoStrength.com**.

Made in the USA
Monee, IL
18 September 2021